S0-ASH-901

HIPPOCRATIC, RELIGIOUS, *and* SECULAR MEDICAL ETHICS

DISCARD

HIPPOCRATIC, RELIGIOUS, *and* SECULAR MEDICAL ETHICS

THE POINTS OF CONFLICT

Robert M. Veatch

GEORGETOWN UNIVERSITY PRESS
Washington, DC

© 2012 Georgetown University Press. All rights reserved. No part of this book may be reproduced or utilized in any form or by any means, electronic or mechanical, including photocopying and recording, or by any information storage and retrieval system, without permission in writing from the publisher.

Library of Congress Cataloging-in-Publication Data

Veatch, Robert M.
  Hippocratic, religious, and secular medical ethics : the points of conflict / Robert M. Veatch.
    p.   cm.
  Includes bibliographical references (p.   ) and index.
  ISBN 978-1-58901-946-1 (pbk. : alk. paper)
    1. Medical ethics.   2. Hippocrates.   3. Medical ethics—Religious aspects—Catholic Church.   I. Title.
  R724.V415   2012
  174.2′2—dc23

                                                              2012019192

♾ This book is printed on acid-free paper meeting the requirements of the American National Standard for Permanence in Paper for Printed Library Materials.

19 18 17 16 15 14 13 12   9 8 7 6 5 4 3 2
First printing

CONTENTS

TABLES

PREFACE AND ACKNOWLEDGMENTS

THIS BOOK HAS DEVELOPED out of my 2008 contribution to the Gifford Lectures, a lecture series that dates back to Scottish lawyer and jurist Adam Lord Gifford's bequest in 1887 establishing funds for lectures at four Scottish universities (Edinburgh, Glasgow, St. Andrews, and Aberdeen). The series, now having taken place for more than 120 years, has itself become something of a phenomenon. No fewer than four books are devoted to the history of the series.[1] The most accessible of these, Larry Witham's *The Measure of God: Our Century-Long Struggle to Reconcile Science & Religion*, carries the subtitle "The Story of the Gifford Lectures." It provides a sweeping history of how Lord Gifford, a senator of the College of Justice of Scotland, culminated his life-long interest in rational understanding of the relation of science to religion and philosophy by leaving a large portion of his estate to create a lecture series. The series was to explore this relation "without reference to or reliance upon any supposed special exceptional or so-called miraculous revelation."[2]

What has followed from this insightful generosity is a series now stretching to more than two hundred lecturers, most of whose Gifford efforts have been published as books. Several of the lecturers have come from philosophy, including William James (*The Varieties of Religious Experience*), Alfred North Whitehead (*Process and Reality*), John Dewey (*The Quest for Certainty*), Ralph Barton Perry (*Realms of Value*), W. D. Ross (*Foundations of Ethics*), and Iris Murdoch (*Metaphysics as a Guide*

ix

to Morals). From theology the lecturers have included Paul Tillich (*Systematic Theology*), Reinhold Niebuhr (*Nature and Destiny of Man*), Karl Barth (*The Knowledge of God and the Service of God*), and Albert Schweitzer. Natural scientists have included Niels Bohr, Werner Heisenberg, and John Eccles. Historian Arnold Toynbee and linguist Noam Chomsky have also appeared.

It has been a privilege and a humbling experience to join in this continuing exploration of the foundations of our natural knowledge of the most fundamental spheres of human existence. When deciding my topic for the series, I naturally turned to the area of my life's work—the ethics of medicine. Knowing that the lecturers were directed by Lord Gifford to focus on "promoting, advancing, teaching, and diffusing the study of natural theology in the widest sense of that term," and realizing that he specifically included "knowledge of the nature and foundations of ethics or morals," I clearly understood that my topic had to be the grounding or the sources of ethics for the professions, especially medicine.[3] Many Gifford lecturers have taken advantage of the invitation to construct a summary of the main themes of their scholarly interest in their careers; I took upon myself the task of exploring the relationship of traditional professionally generated medical ethics to the primary sources of ethics outside the professions, that is, to philosophy and religion. Many laypeople and medical professionals associate professional medical ethics with the Hippocratic Oath and the tradition surrounding that document. I decided to focus on the points of conflict between Hippocratic medical ethics and the ethics rooted in religious and secular philosophical traditions. My major effort would be to profess the inadequacies of the Hippocratic tradition (or any other professional ethic that claims its origins from within a professional group).

In contracting my analysis of the grounding of ethical claims for the professions, I needed examples of different moral epistemologies. It was natural in the context of the Giffords that in some cases I turned to previous lecturers for these illustrations. Thus, I turned to Karl Barth and Stanley Hauerwas as two of the most profound defenders of revelation as a source of moral knowledge—that is, as proponents of nonnatural moral epistemologies. I would have chosen them regardless of their connection with the Giffords. I also relied on others who have not been contributors to the lecture series, including the fascinating case of Oral Roberts and the more complex cases of Judaism and H. Tristram Engelhardt, a proponent of Eastern Orthodoxy. When I turned to natural religious epistemologies, I relied on illustrations unrelated to the Giffords: mainstream Roman Catholicism as well as three Protestant examples: Philipp Melancthon, John Calvin, and John Wesley. These three were meant to illustrate positions widely recognized within religious ethics.

Likewise, when I turned to secular philosophy, I included Ralph Barton Perry and (in chapter 7) W. D. Ross—both former Gifford lecturers, but they are also among the most influential figures in twentieth-century moral philosophy, and most of my examples come from the mainstream of philosophical ethics—Kant, Rawls, the philosophers of the Scottish Enlightenment, and some of the main theorists in bioethics—who have not been involved with the Giffords. Nevertheless, they illustrate the concerns that Lord Gifford had about ways of knowing, which become central to my project of identifying tensions between professional sources of knowing, on the one hand, and religious and philosophical sources, on the other.

Relatively few previous Gifford lecturers have focused on medicine. William James trained as a physician, but his contributions focus on philosophy, psychology, and religion. Famed neurophysiologists Charles Sherrington and John Eccles presented lectures in the 1930s and 1970s; more recently, philosopher-bioethicist Onora O'Neill discussed the concept of autonomy and trust in bioethics, but no one has ever taken on the problem of the grounding of professional ethics and the relation of professional to religious and secular philosophical sources. That would become my topic.

Although publication of the lectures as a book is the norm, the Gifford committee does not enter into the lecturer's relation with publishers. This allows authors time after the lectures to make revisions and additions and to work with publishers. I have taken advantage of the time since my days in Edinburgh to rework and expand my research and have now developed that work into this volume. Thus, this book has been in the works for about a decade, counting the years prior to the lecture presentation in 2008 and the years expanding and crafting the manuscript since that time.

I am grateful to Sir Timothy O'Shea, the principal and vice chancellor of the University of Edinburgh and the convener of the Gifford Lectureships Committee, and to Stewart Brown of the School of Divinity, the deputy convener, for their generous invitation to be the Gifford lecturer for 2008. I am also indebted to Isabel Roberts, the secretary to the committee, for her gracious and efficient handling of the details of my visit to Edinburgh. I had previously spent my 1996 sabbatical at the Institute for Advanced Studies in the Humanities at the university, so my return there was a particularly welcome experience. I thank Susan Manning, director of the institute, for her hospitality during my return visit. I am grateful to groups at Georgetown University, Washington and Lee University, Haverford College, and the University of Otago in New Zealand for opportunities to try out aspects of the arguments in this volume prior to my time at Edinburgh. I am also grateful to my friend and colleague James Drane, who hosted a gathering of the "Founders of Bioethics" in June of 2010, which gave me a further opportunity to try out some of my ideas for this project with Jim and many of the others of bioethics' founding generation. Plans are under way to publish those conversations at some future point.

Much of the research for the Gifford and for this book was done from my base of the last thirty years at the Kennedy Institute of Ethics at Georgetown University. I have been blessed with an appointment that gives me enormous freedom to pursue topics of interest. My appointment also gives me a wonderful group of colleagues, including the world's best group of professional bioethics librarians at the institute's bioethics research library. For their help on countless scholarly and technical research questions and in tracking down obscure sources, I owe them much. Philosophy graduate student Yashar Saghai was particularly helpful in providing research assistance, especially in dealing with French,

Arabic, and Muslim sources. Kennedy Institute of Ethics intern Matthew Westbrook and research assistant Samantha Thompson contributed research as well.

I am very pleased to be publishing this book with the press of my home university. The press's director, Richard Brown, has been a friend and colleague for many years, and I have grown to admire his knowledge of publishing in ethics, especially bioethics. His interest in and support of this volume has been a pleasure and inspiration. I am honored to have had the cooperation of someone whose publishing and substantive knowledge of the field I admire.

My wife Ann made the trip to Edinburgh with me and tolerated the years of pursuit of sometimes absurdly troublesome questions. She remains my strength in all I do in life.

INTRODUCTION
The Hippocratic Problem

HE HIPPOCRATIC OATH often commands the status of a timeless, universal moral code for physicians and other health practitioners. A widespread assumption exists that the Oath is an
uncontroversial moral code for the practice of medicine at any time or
place under which physicians pledge that they will always work for the
benefit of the patient and protect the patient from harm. While that is
the Hippocratic pledge, this pledge occupies a status far from the harm-
less platitude often assigned to it. In this book I reexamine the Hippocratic Oath and, more generally, professional ethics in the Hippocratic
tradition to explore their relation to various religious and secular ethical
codes for health care. I conclude that the Oath is so controversial and
so offensive that it can no longer stand alongside religious and secular
alternatives. I argue that the Hippocratic Oath is unacceptable to any
thinking person. It should offend the patient and challenge any health
care professional to look elsewhere for moral authority.

I argue that the Hippocratic Oath reflects the ethic of an ancient
Greek cult (and not a very sophisticated one at that). It necessarily stands
in conflict with any of the other religious ethical systems of the world,
including all the major religions, and with any secular ethical tradition
as well. I claim that a physician can be a member of a major religious

1

tradition—Jewish, Catholic, or Methodist, for example—or can be a Hippocratist, but not both, at least not both simultaneously. I claim that a physician can be a practitioner of any of the major secular traditions—a liberal pluralist, a Marxist, or a libertarian, for example—or a Hippocratist, but not both. I also examine whether, if one abandons the Hippocratic medical-ethical tradition in favor of some more plausible alternative, one can simultaneously commit to a religious ethic and a secular moral system. I suggest that the "natural theology" designated by Adam Lord Gifford to be the focus of the Gifford Lectures is critical to this question, that at least if one accepts some role for reason and experience or for a "common morality," religious and secular medical ethics are compatible with each other but not with the Hippocratic ethic. To be sure, revealed religious ethics remains in greater tension with its secular analogues, but, so I shall claim, religious ethics based on natural means of knowing are potentially compatible with secular ethics. Nevertheless, any plausible religious or secular medical ethical system must stand in inevitable conflict with the ethic that derives from the Hippocratic Oath.

A helpful reviewer of a draft of this volume was critical of my attack on the Hippocratic Oath not because she wanted to defend it but rather because she was aware that contemporary bioethics scholars have sometimes recognized the Oath's inadequacies. She was aware, as I shall document in detail, that the Oath has been replaced as a moral guide for medical professional groups and for medical school graduation rituals.

I must make two points. First, while some scholars are aware of the Hippocratic Oath's limits, more popular culture and most professionals within medicine still treat the Oath as if it were the foundation of their moral relation with patients. For example, the American Medical Association has started its *Code of Medical Ethics* for many years with reference to the Hippocratic Oath. It begins, "The Oath of Hippocrates, a brief statement of principles, has come down through history as a living statement of ideals to be cherished by the physician." It goes on to say that the Oath "protected the rights of the patient and appealed to the inner and finer instincts of the physician." Further, the Oath "has remained in Western civilization as an expression of ideal conduct for the physician."[1]

The same words have appeared in every edition of the AMA's *Code* for at least three decades. Nowhere does the AMA recognize the tension between the Hippocratic Oath and the more plausible modern principles it articulates. Similarly, the British Medical Association acknowledges the Hippocratic Oath as the foundation of physician ethics, saying, "The Hippocratic Oath and its successors, such as the World Medical Association's Declaration of Geneva, have expressed a fundamental medical duty to pursue patients' best medical interests, to avoid harming or exploiting them, and to maintain their confidences."[2] I could cite countless examples of medical professionals and their organizations appealing to the Oath in spite of its many flaws.

Similarly, lawyers, judges, and expert witnesses often appeal to the Oath when attempting to establish the ethical or legal duties of physicians. Steven Shafer, the star prosecution witness in the trial of Michael Jackson's physician, Conrad Murray, said that Murray violated his Hippocratic Oath, which, he said, has held doctors to high standards since ancient times.[3] The lawyer for the Jackson family said, erroneously, that physicians cannot "cast aside their Hippocratic oath to do no harm,"[4] apparently believing that Dr. Murray had at some point actually taken the Hippocratic Oath and had pledged to "do no harm." In the sentencing, Judge Michael Pastor repeated the accusation, saying Murray "violated his obligations to his patient in the essence of his Hippocratic Oath."[5]

More significantly, even some contemporary bioethics scholars still attribute moral authority to the Oath. For example, Steven Miles's volume *The Hippocratic Oath and the Ethics of Medicine* provides a more nuanced approach but still ends up concluding that "the Oath can serve as an attractive and serviceable framework for a modern medical ethics curriculum rather than simply being relegated to ritualistic history."[6] Many texts and casebooks in medical ethics include the Hippocratic Oath as one, or perhaps the only, codification for study. In at least two places the well-known volume by Albert Jonsen, Mark Siegler, and William Winslade, *Clinician Ethics: A Practical Approach to Ethical*

Decisions in Clinical Medicine, cites the Hippocratic Oath without qualification, as if it were the legitimate basis for determining moral norms
for physicians.[7] A recent collection of essays, *Ethical Dilemmas in Pediatrics*, is introduced with the platitudinous (and factually incorrect) statement that "physicians, nurses, and hospital administrators all operate
under professional codes which are 'Hippocratic.'"[8] This literature does
not take seriously the possibility that, in principle, professionally generated oaths and codes are no longer an acceptable basis for medical
morality.

I offer a second point in response to the suggestion that the Hippocratic Oath is no longer considered the morally definitive code of ethics
for physicians. While the substantive normative ethical principles of the
Oath are challenged in this volume, far more important is my claim that
the metaethics of not only the Oath but of all professionally generated
codes of ethics must be called into question. Metaethics deals with the
means of justifying an ethic and its foundational authority. This volume
challenges the presumption that professional groups have the authority
to promulgate codes of ethics for their members. Thus, not only the
Hippocratic Oath, generated by a group of physicians in ancient Greece,
but also all codes written by medical professional organizations—in fact,
by organizations of any profession—need to be examined to see if the
authority of professionals to establish the moral norms for their group is
legitimate. I argue that it is not. After one acknowledges that the Hippocratic Oath is ethically unacceptable, one must press on to determine if
the alternative codifications produced by modern professional groups are
any more defensible. I argue that they are not.

Before launching this exploration, let me make clear what I mean by
professional ethics. The term is systematically ambiguous, which can
cause considerable confusion. Professional ethics has something to do
with ethics as it involves the professions, no doubt. I will concentrate on
the health professions, especially the profession of the physician, but
what I have to say applies to all the health professions and even other
professions—the law, the ministry, the academic, the accountancy—as
well.

The term "professional ethics" can be used to refer to ethics formulated, articulated, and enforced by a professional group. As such, it surely deals with the conduct of the members of the profession, but the term can also refer to ethical pronouncements by the group about the conduct of others, especially the clients of the professional. Hence, the original American Medical Association code of ethics has an entire section on the obligations of patients toward physicians. For example, the fifth provision of the section's ten provisions on the obligations of patients to their physicians holds that "a patient should never weary his physician with a tedious detail of events or matters not appertaining to his disease. Even as relates to his actual symptoms, he will convey much more real information by giving clear answers to interrogatories, than by the most minute account of his own framing."[9] The moral requirement imposed on patients continues: "The obedience of a patient to the prescriptions of his physician should be prompt and implicit. He should never permit his own crude opinions as to their fitness to influence his attention to them."[10] I will refer to these codes written by professional groups as professionally generated or articulated ethics.

Not all professional ethics is professionally generated or articulated. Other individuals and groups comment from time to time about the ethical conduct of professionals. Religious groups, for example, may generate codes that stipulate the way they think physicians should act—that they should refuse to perform abortions or should spend a certain portion of their time caring for the poor, for example. Thus, groups outside the profession can comment on professional conduct, and this could be called "professional ethics" as well. Of course, these groups may also offer comments on the moral conduct of laypeople, such as members of the religion, when they interact with professionals. A church (or a government or a philosopher) that said it would be immoral for a patient to ask a professional to help the patient commit suicide would be offering a pronouncement about ethics as it impacts the professional, but this would be neither a professionally generated ethic nor an ethic about the conduct of the professional. I am interested in this volume in the justification of professionally generated or articulated ethics and how these relate to pronouncements from outside the professional group about the conduct of professionals and the patients with whom professionals interact.

One further distinction is critical. The observation that either professional or nonprofessional groups may generate codifications about professional conduct needs to be kept separate from claims about whether there can be special duties for members of a professional group. There can be "role-specific duties," duties attached to specific roles—professional, familial, or interpersonal—that require people in certain roles to act in unique and different ways from what is normally required of people outside these roles. Police or soldiers may shoot people with guns in ways that are totally unacceptable for people who are not police or soldiers. Parents may show partiality toward their children that would be inexcusable for teachers or those in other roles. Possibly CIA agents may tell lies in ways not permitted by the normal rules of veracity.

I believe it is indisputable that health professionals have certain role-specific duties. They must remain loyal to patients in ways unnecessary for those in many other roles—they must stay on duty during a plague or flood, for example. Physicians in the military have duties toward the enemy combatant that are radically different from the duties of those they serve alongside. Health professionals are also granted certain privileges—for example, to probe intimately and cut open a body.

When I question whether professionally generated codes of ethics are legitimate or whether ethics for a profession must be grounded in more general religious or secular normative ethical systems, I am not disputing the claim that these general religious or secular normative systems may affirm special duties for those in special roles including professional roles. I am claiming that the professional group cannot be the source of these special duties, that the role-specific duties must be derived from those ethical norms that have their foundation outside the profession, and must be comprehensible to reasonable laypeople who are outside the professional group. Thus, just as someone who is not a police officer may understand and accept that police officers have special rights and duties regarding the shooting of people, so someone who is not a physician may understand and accept that physicians have special rights and duties in a natural disaster.

I begin in chapter 1 with the grandfather of professionally generated codes, the Hippocratic Oath. After offering some analysis of the Oath itself, I broaden my inquiry in chapter 2 to other professionally generated ethical pronouncements. Chapter 3 zeros in on the role of medical schools and professional associations in transmitting professional codes of ethics to medical students and other initiates into the profession. I note the oddity that different schools and associations inflict different codifications, sometimes with significantly different moral requirements, on their newly minted members of the profession even though these students and new physicians will practice together in hospitals and group practices, leaving patients and other professionals to figure out how those who have made diverse ethical pledges should interact in the care of their patients. I also note the strangeness of taking student enrollees who no doubt hold diverse moral views about medical practices such as abortion, euthanasia, consent, and confidentiality and imposing on them a single, uniform code that cannot possibly square with the views of each of the students. For example, the imposed code at St. George's University School of Medicine (where I have taught medical ethics for the past twenty-three years) has its students swear in the name of God despite the fact that at least one troubled and puzzled student of mine confessed she was an atheist and did not know whether she should pledge in the name of the deity in which she had no faith. I sort out these puzzles and argue that physicians and medical students should never be asked to pledge to a one-size-fits-all code prepackaged for them.

Chapter 4 summarizes the case against professionally generated codes of ethics for a profession. I focus on the health professions and medicine in particular, but the argument applies to any professional group. I note that some professionally generated codes impose very strange moral requirements on the group's members, and that it is common for a professional group to have generated more than one code of ethics. Sometimes these codes are contradictory, so a member of the profession must violate one of the professional codes in order to follow another. I then take up the "internal morality of medicine" thesis in which it is claimed—erroneously, I suggest—that the very concept of a profession such as medicine contains within it normative content that sets the moral norms for its practitioners. I then close the chapter with three examples (withholding nutrition from terminal patients, physician participation in capital punishment, and surrogate motherhood) in which professionally generated codes seem to pose insurmountable problems.

Chapter 5 turns to religious ethics as an alternative source of morality, including morality for the practice of medicine. In contrast with professional associations, I concede that religions can be, in principle, a legitimate source of moral norms. That is to say, for those who believe in a particular theology, it makes sense for them to hold that moral obligations have their roots in the most foundational beliefs of their tradition. This, I claim, is not true in the case of a profession. Whether a particular religious tradition can plausibly hold that its religious moral norms are legitimate for relations between patient and professional when at least one of those parties is not a member of the religious group is, I argue, dependent on whether the religion sees its norms as revealed, as knowable only through what Lord Gifford would consider "nonnatural" means of knowing or, alternatively, whether it sees the norms as knowable through reason or experience in principle accessible to all human beings—Lord Gifford's natural ways of knowing.

That sets the stage for chapter 6, in which I turn to secular philosophical ways of knowing moral norms and whether they are compatible with the more theological ways of knowing that appropriately dominate professionals and laypeople who see themselves inside one or another of the religious traditions. I argue that secular ways of knowing moral norms are shared by all human beings, and that these ways of knowing through reason, experience, and what is in contemporary bioethical theory called "common morality" are equally accessible to medical professionals and medical laypeople. Finally, in chapter 7 I bring together my discussion of religious and secular sources of medical ethics, proposing what I call a "convergence hypothesis." I claim that, after taking into account the limits imposed by human fallibility, this common morality is shared by religious theorists who are willing to accept natural ways of knowing their theological insights (even if they are incapable of communication with revealed ethical systems). It is these religious/secular sources—what Lord Gifford would have considered "natural" sources—that must provide the foundation for medical ethics and the ethical obligations of health professionals and laypeople. Rather than professionally generated or articulated codes of ethics, this foundation must underpin the morality of lay–professional relations in medicine. Two kinds of issues might concern someone about professionally generated codes. First, one might be concerned about the substance of the ethical positions—the normative ethics, to use the technical term. A professionally generated code could oppose, for example, physician participation in abortion or could endorse the duty of the physician to keep all information about a patient confidential. Some normative positions such as these might be controversial. One who believes some abortions are moral and that physicians should assist patients who obtain them would reject a professionally generated moral code that opposes abortion. One who believes that doctors sometimes have a duty to breach confidentiality in order to warn nonpatients who are in imminent danger from a patient would similarly reject a professionally generated moral code that mandates confidentiality in these circumstances.

Second, and in some ways more important, someone might be concerned about how the profession claims to know what is morally right or wrong for a member of its organization or why it claims to be authoritative in pronouncing about the morality of the conduct of its members (and occasionally even shows the hubris of pronouncing on moral duties for patients and other nonmembers). These are problems of moral epistemology—ways of knowing—that are independent of the normative claims of a professional ethic. These are problems of metaethics.

CHAPTER

1

THE HIPPOCRATIC OATH
AND THE ETHIC OF
HIPPOCRATISM

REGARDLESS OF THE modern widespread acceptance of the Hippocratic Oath as an uncontroversial, platitudinous statement with universal application, its origins are more eccentric. It is associated with the Hippocratic school of medicine in ancient Greece, one among many competing medical schools of thought. Its adherents came up against the Empiricists, Rationalists, Methodists, and Asclepions. The Hippocratic school, sometimes referred to as the Coan school, was apparently centered on the island of Cos in the Aegean Sea, far removed from mainland Greece and some four kilometers from the Turkish coast.[1]

The Oath was, in all likelihood, not written by a historical figure named Hippocrates but more likely by one of his followers some decades after the death of the teacher for whom the school is named. This would place the Oath in the fourth century before the common era.[2] For our purposes, it is critical to understand that the Oath reflects characteristics that suggest an initiation ritual into a kind of Greek cult. Ludwig Edelstein, the twentieth-century German physician-historian, sees the group responsible for the Oath as Pythagorean.[3] The Pythagoreans were a quasi-religious, scientific, mathematical, and philosophical group that reflected many of the characteristics of the Oath, including its tripartite division of medicine into dietetics, pharmacology, and surgery. Scholarship since the eighteenth century has proposed that the Oath could be Pythagorean.[4]

More recent scholarship has questioned the Pythagorean hypothesis put forward by Edelstein and his predecessors.[5] Some claim that all that can be said is that the Oath represents the thinking of a group with some characteristics resembling the Pythagoreans. We need not resolve this dispute. The origin is either from a Pythagorean group or from a group that is in many ways similar. To avoid taking sides in this scholarly feud, I refer to the Hippocratic cultic group as "Pythagorean-like." Regardless of how that dispute is resolved, the critical point is that the Hippocratic Oath represents the moral and religious views of one particular group with a rather special view of how medicine should be practiced. Only by crude, simplistic, reductionist maneuvers can the unique and peculiar characteristics of the Hippocratic Oath be extended to an all-purpose, universal codification for the proper moral conduct of all physicians.

My focus is not primarily on the original meaning and content of the Oath as used by some ancient pagan religious school of physicians, whoever they may have been, but on the use of the Oath as a codification of moral norms for health care professionals in the modern world. In criticizing the moral content of the Oath as a source of guidance for modern physicians, my aim is not to suggest it was inappropriate for the group practicing Hippocratic medicine in ancient Greece. Rather, I am saying the Oath is seriously deficient for dealing with the medical morality of the present day. I argue that it is incompatible with both modern secular ethical systems and major religious traditions of contemporary medical morality.

The Normative Peculiarities of the Oath

The peculiarities and religious uniqueness of the Oath as a source relevant to modern medical practice are apparent in the first line, even if that line provides only the most superficial problems for modern medical practitioners. The Oath begins by having the physician swear by "Apollo the Physician and Asclepius and Hygieia and Panaceia and all the gods and goddesses."[6] Already the Oath text should give the modern physician (and layperson) pause. In its classic form, the Oath is not only a religious document; it is one of a pagan Greek religion that should offend the practitioner as well as the patient of any modern religious or secular persuasion.

Almost all modern versions of the Oath edit out the embarrassing pagan deities. In doing so, however, they erase the initial signal that the Oath is grounded in a religious alternative to the views of virtually all modern health providers and patients. Moreover, cleansing the Oath of its most explicit religious references merely masks the more subtle problems buried in the text.

The Peculiar Oath of Initiation

The Oath is divided into two main sections: a pledge of loyalty resembling an initiation oath and a code of conduct. Greek medicine involved transmission of the knowledge of the practice to members of a clan. It is possible that those outside the group would swear an oath signifying their adoption into the group. The initiation section requires the physician to pledge to hold his teachers as equal to his parents. It goes so far as to extract a promise that if the teacher is ever in need of money, the initiate will give him a share of the student's resources. He will regard the teacher's offspring as "brothers in male lineage" who will in turn be taught the art of medicine without fee. Something akin to what modern universities call a "legacy" seems to exist. The children of the teacher deserve a special "scholarship" outside the normal means of entering the cult. The exact meaning of these provisions and the context in which the Oath was administered have been lost to history. Disputes exist over whether there was ever a formal "adoption" ceremony by which medical students were incorporated into the family of the Hippocratic cult. The surviving language, however, is sufficient to signal that some rather peculiar ritual was involved, one that surely does not fit modern medicine. The thought that the modern physician would somehow be adopted into a "family" of practitioners should be alienating to modern patients.

The Peculiar Code of Ethics

After extracting a promise that the initiate will not divulge the secrets of the cult, the Oath then moves into the moral code section. Applying the three-part division of medicine, the Oath has the physician give first priority to dietetics, a division and priority that suggests similarity to Pythagorean thought. It is here that the core Hippocratic moral insight first appears. The physician pledges, "I will apply dietetic measures for the benefit of the sick according to my ability and judgment; I will keep them from harm and injustice."[7] While this commitment might at first seem uncontroversial, it is in fact interpreted, at least in modern medical ethics, to require potentially offensive behavior of the physician in at least three ways.

First, it ignores nonconsequentialistic moral norms found in Kantian ethics, systems of religious moral law, other duty-based traditions, and the tradition of human rights. For example, in certain interesting cases, a physician may face a conflict between respecting the rights of a patient and doing what the physician believes will benefit the patient. Treating a terminally ill patient against her consent is an example. Hippocratic physicians have long recognized cases in which disclosure of information to a patient about diagnosis, prognosis, or potential therapies might do harm to the patient, for instance, by causing psychological distress. This suggests another example of the conflict between doing what the physician believes will benefit the patient and respecting the rights of the patient. Following the mandate to always act to benefit the patient and protect the patient from harm, Hippocratic physicians have felt morally obliged to withhold such information. The idea is often referred to as a "therapeutic privilege." The physician is believed to have the privilege of acting "therapeutically," dispensing information as other therapies only when "medically indicated."[8] This practice conflicts with the basic right of a patient to be informed about therapy and to give consent before being treated. Since nonconsequentialistic rights and duties such as the principle of respect for autonomy are absent from the Hippocratic ethic, no intrinsic duty to inform and obtain consent is present in the ethic derived from the Oath.

Second, the commitment to benefit the patient and keep the patient from harm and injustice puts forth a paternalistic standard of determining what will benefit patients. It is the physician's own judgment rather than the views of some broader, more objective moral community or of the patients themselves that forms the basis for deciding what will benefit patients.[9] Thus, not only are rights and duties subordinated to patient benefit, but patient benefit is also determined by the odd standard of the individual physician's judgment.

Third, and perhaps most critically, the Hippocratic principle of benefiting the patient ignores the possibility of a social ethics in which physicians might have the right or duty to sacrifice their patients for the good of others in society. The rigorous Hippocratic standard focusing exclusively on benefit for the patient requires abandoning any moral concerns for anyone beyond the patient. These can arise in matters such as public health, human subjects research, and resource allocation. While Jewish and Christian ethics are nothing if not social or communitarian, and modern secular ethics normally incorporates theories of aggregate social utility maximizing or of distributive justice, or both, the Hippocratic norm is devoid of any of these.

In its core Hippocratic principle of benefiting the patient and protecting the patient from harm according to the physician's judgment, the Oath puts forward a very peculiar moral norm, one devoid of moral principles other than promoting benefit and avoiding harm, one that gives pride of place to the physician's judgments to the exclusion of those of others, and one that ignores the possibility of a social moral duty.[10] In all of these characteristics, the Oath is diametrically opposed to most major religious and secular ethical stances. In fact, it can be argued that no other ethical theory in the history of the world's religious and secular moral traditions has ever combined these peculiar characteristics. My point is not necessarily that such an ethic was inappropriate for ancient Greek culture. Establishing that would require more work. Rather, my point is that such an ethic is laughingly deficient for any modern religious or secular worldview.

Physicians, then, must choose. They can be Hippocratists or Christians, Hippocratists or members of some other religious tradition, but they cannot simultaneously be members of the Hippocratic cult and some other religion with competing moral stances. They can be Hippocratists or Kantians, Hippocratists or classical utilitarians, Hippocratists or members of some other secular tradition, but they cannot simultaneously be members of the Hippocratic tradition and some other secular tradition with competing moral stances. The strangeness of the ethical code of the Hippocratic Oath, at least for modern medical practice, becomes more evident when one examines the line-by-line commitments one makes in swearing the Hippocratic pledge.

Giving Deadly Drugs   The section on dietetics is followed by some ethical norms dealing with pharmacology—that is, the use of drugs, the second tier of the tripartite division of Hippocratic medicine. It begins by having the Hippocratic physician pledge, "I will neither give a deadly drug to anybody if asked for it, nor will I make a suggestion to this effect."[11] In modern interpretations, this is usually understood as a prohibition on physician participation in euthanasia. Although taken literally, it seems to prohibit only drugs that are deadly; other nonpharmacological methods are normally included by extension. From this, physicians deduce not only a prohibition on physician participation in executions but also on physician administration of drugs that hasten death in the terminally ill and suffering, sometimes called active euthanasia.[12]

Some have seen this as evidence of compatibility between Hippocratic ethics and a Christian ethics that opposes killing. They suggest that early Christians in the post-Constantinian world could not accept other Greek and Roman traditions that endorsed merciful killings, so, during the Christianization of Rome, the Hippocratic ethic for medicine was elevated to a higher, more acceptable status.[13] As we shall see, there is precious little evidence for this hypothesis and good reason to reject it. Nevertheless, the prohibition on physician killing is a feature of the Hippocratic Oath that deserves attention.

Some modern physicians have recognized the potential tension between the duty to do what the physician believes will benefit the patient and the duty to avoid giving deadly drugs. American physician Jack Kevorkian concluded that when the two clash, the more fundamental requirement is to benefit the patient.[14] His explicit utilitarianism, when applied to suffering patients, led him to conclude he had a duty to benefit patients by assisting in their suicides. In at least one case, he extended this to the active killing of a patient by lethal injection on grounds of mercy. In an attempt to be benevolent, Kevorkian murdered an ALS patient who was physically unable to commit suicide, which led to Kevorkian's conviction and imprisonment.[15]

The more traditional interpretation of the Hippocratic prohibition on giving a deadly drug reaches a different conclusion. Giving deadly drugs is seen as always contrary to a patient's interest, thus avoiding the potential conflict between the two injunctions of the Oath. On the other hand, the citizens of the Netherlands and of the American states of Oregon, Washington, and Montana have concluded that the old Hippocratic cult was wrong on this issue.[16] The Netherlands policy permits the giving of deadly drugs, and the American policies permit recommending and prescribing them but not administering them. Their citizens have thus rejected (or ignored) the Oath's injunction. Because the lay citizens of these jurisdictions are not supposed to be capable of comprehending the Hippocratic injunction, this deviation would be understandable. The misalignment, however, presents a more serious problem for physicians who claim to be Hippocratic.

Abortive Remedies   The next subject of the pharmacological section of the Oath prohibits giving a woman an "abortive remedy." The Greek term is often interpreted as referring to "abortive pessary," a vaginal suppository that was a standard method of inducing abortion. This provision has caused considerable concern for moderns. Those who are more liberal on abortion have tried to claim that this merely prohibits a single abortion method, freeing up physicians to use all modern techniques. On the other hand, conservatives on abortion have sometimes recognized their need to go beyond the Hippocratic restriction on the single pessary method.

The prohibitions on giving deadly drugs and on abortion are cited by Edelstein as grounds for connecting the Hippocratic Oath with Pythagoreanism.[17] Although neither euthanasia nor abortion was condemned in most Greek thought, they were violations to the Pythagoreans. Whether these were ethical problems for Pythagoreans or other Greek schools of thought should be, of course, irrelevant to those whose ethics come from other religious or secular traditions. The point for our purposes is that the Oath's peculiar condemnation of giving a pessary to produce an abortion can be seen as odd—indeed, problematic—to modern people probing the ethics of abortion. It may not even be the case that the giving of the pessary was condemned because of moral doubts about abortion at all. Kudlien suggests that the Oath writer's objection may have something to do with an "odium of strong 'uncleanness,'" that is, ritual impurity, which has been associated in some ancient cultures with the practice of abortion.[18] If so, the Hippocratic provision would be quite irrelevant to moderns unconcerned about such spiritual defilement.

The Virtues of Purity and Holiness   The Oath concludes the pharmacological section by introducing the two virtues of the Hippocratic school: purity and holiness. These are striking and indeed should be problematic for moderns as well as for most Greeks. The classic Platonic virtues—wisdom, temperance, justice, and courage—would seem to put forth very different character ideals than these more religiously tainted norms. Even for the religiously inclined, these virtues are controversial. They differ from the classic Christian theological virtues of faith, hope, and charity.

The terms "purity" and "holiness" have a religious aura about them. Their precise meaning has been the subject of much contemporary scholarship.[19] Surely, "holiness" is undeniably a religious term. "Purity" should be seen that way as well. The term is widely recognized as conveying a norm for being ritually clean. Many archaic tribal religions insist that their priestly class be ritually pure. This includes a requirement of ritual cleaning after contamination with defiling substances such as blood. Hence, priests (*Kohanim*) in Judaism are not permitted to engage in ritual sacrifice. Edelstein cites these virtues of purity and holiness as being consistent with Pythagorean thought, although they certainly are also consistent with a much broader spectrum of Greek beliefs.[20]

The Prohibition on Surgery   The concern about ritual defilement from contact with blood provides the only plausible explanation for the odd provision condemning the participation of the Hippocratic physician in surgery. The prohibition on surgery is an embarrassing puzzle for modern medical students, especially those contemplating surgical specialization. They usually simply ignore it.

Some attempt to rationalize the prohibition by pointing out that, in the era before germ theory, a wise physician would come to know that surgery would inevitably lead to contamination and serious consequences, or they see it as an injunction not to go beyond one's area of medical competence.[21] This would provide an explanation for a prohibition on surgery that was correct in Hippocratic times but irrelevant in the era of aseptic technique.

The problem with that rationalization of the Hippocratic prohibition is that the Oath goes on to state that the Hippocratic physician should leave surgery to "such men as are engaged in this work," that is, other practitioners who are not part of the Hippocratic group. That would make no sense if the Hippocratist believed that surgery should be eschewed because of the danger of infection.

The most plausible speculation is that Hippocratists were physicians who understood their role in ritualistic religious terms. They were priestly practitioners who had a special duty to avoid blood contamination even though such contact with blood would not pose the same problem for those standing outside the priestly role.[22] Concerns about ritual defilement, especially impurity from contact with blood, were very common in traditional cultures. The issue comes up in ancient Judaism and many traditional cultures, including the Greek and Roman.

Abstaining from Sexual Relations with Patients and Patients' Family Members   The next paragraph of the Oath is sometimes cited as the basis for the professional norm that prohibits sexual relations with patients. The text repeats the controversial Hippocratic norm that the physician, when entering houses, will come for the benefit of the sick, "remaining free of all intentional injustice, of all mischief and in particular of sexual relations with both female and male persons, be they free or slaves." While moderns see this as a prohibition on sexual relations with patients, ancients might have noticed in particular the application to both genders and to slaves as well as free. Surely, no modern ethic would go out of its way to emphasize that it is both men and women, both slave and free, who should not be the target of the physician's sexual interest.

Confidentiality   Next the Oath introduces what is usually taken as a central idea in medical ethics but one that is presented in a strikingly controversial way in the Hippocratic text. It states: "What I may see or hear in the course of the treatment or even outside of the treatment in regard to the life of men, which on no account one must spread abroad, I will keep to myself holding such things shameful to be spoken about."[23] Modern rights-based theories of confidentiality require that the physician keep the patient's information confidential unless the patient allows disclosure. By contrast, the standard Hippocratic position not only permits but actually requires the physician to disclose such information if the physician believes the disclosure would benefit the patient—even if the patient insists that the information not be disclosed.

This is the mainstream paternalistic interpretation. It was the position taken by the British General Medical Council in the 1970 British case of a Dr. Brown who learned that his sixteen-year-old patient was on the birth control pill.[24] Dr. Brown believed that this was not good for her and felt morally obliged to tell her father. When Dr. Brown was charged with a breach of confidentiality, he cited the Hippocratic Oath (as well as the British and American medical association codes of ethics) in his defense and was acquitted of any violation. He had disclosed only because he believed, according to his judgment, that disclosure would be beneficial to his patient. Thus, he was acting in accord with the Oath, which was interpreted as prohibiting only those disclosures that "ought not to be spoken abroad." Disclosing information that served the patient's interest was not prohibited according to this paternalistic interpretation of the Oath's clause.

As a result of this case, the British and American codes of ethics were changed to prohibit such paternalistic disclosures. The Hippocratic Oath, at least in its standard interpretation, was morally intolerable in a world in which those in fiduciary roles were not permitted to breach confidences simply because they believed it would serve their patients' interest. The physician cannot disclose because he or she believes it would benefit the patient any more than a priest can disclose the words of the confessional because of a belief that the penitent would benefit. Only with patient permission could such patient-benefiting disclosure be made.

There is an alternative interpretation that requires keeping all patient information confidential no matter the implications. That leaves the physician vulnerable to failing to meet the legal requirement of a duty to warn third parties of threats of potential serious harm. A decade after the Dr. Brown case, another change in the Oath's confidentiality provision was recognized to be necessary. A college student named Prosenjit Poddar was romantically involved with a girl named Tatiana Tarasoff. Before leaving for a semester outside the United States, Tatiana indicated she wanted to break off the relationship. Poddar was so distraught that he sought psychological counseling at the student health service. During this counseling, he confessed that his anger led him to want to kill Tarasoff when she returned to school. The psychologist took him seriously and reported the incident to the campus police, who said they could take no action based on the mere threat. After Tarasoff returned to campus,

Poddar killed her, which led her parents to argue that the health professional had a duty to warn her or her parents of the credible threat. The California courts eventually concluded that the health professional did indeed have a duty to warn, and that the refusal of the police to take action did not absolve him of that duty.[25] Today many legal jurisdictions recognize such a duty.

It might be argued that the only reason that the health professional should warn a potential victim is to protect the perpetrator—that is, the patient of the health professional—who would avoid the risk of serious legal and psychological problems if he were prevented from committing the homicide. If that were the reason, it would be consistent with Hippocratic paternalism. The health professional would be acting for the benefit of the patient (even though that patient may not agree and may not approve). It seems obvious, however, that the real reason the health professional has a duty to breach confidentiality is not to protect the patient but rather to protect that patient's potential victim. The reason is not Hippocratic at all. It is not motivated out of a duty to serve the patient but rather to serve the very real, critical interests of the potential victim.

This view has now been adopted by the American Medical Association in a decision that rejects the Hippocratic reason for breaching confidentiality (patient welfare) and replaces it with a non-Hippocratic reason (the welfare of a third party).[26] Today virtually all medical ethics break with Hippocratic reasoning on confidentiality in favor of a more social ethic that requires, under certain limited and defined conditions, health professionals to act not for the welfare of the patient, but rather for the welfare of others who may be the patient's intended victims. This is one more example of how no reasonable modern ethical system for medicine can follow the Hippocratic model.

The Hippocratic text is deceptively complex and open to at least controversial interpretations. One interpretation reads the clause referring to items "which on no account one must spread abroad" as a restrictive clause. It would be more grammatically correct, then, to translate this into English as referring to "what one sees or hears . . . *that* on no account one must spread abroad." Some translations offer this reading. Unfortunately, Edelstein, whose translation we are using, does not pick up on the important difference depending on whether the "no account" clause is restrictive or nonrestrictive. If read as a restrictive clause, the text implies that only those things that should not be spread abroad should be held as confidential. This, of course, raises the question of what things ought to be spoken abroad. The standard Hippocratic answer introduces the Hippocratic principle here. If the physician has information about the patient, the disclosure of which would benefit the patient, then the physician should disclose; otherwise, the information should be kept confidential.

The second interpretation is to treat the clause as nonrestrictive. In this reading everything seen or heard regarding patients is to be kept confidential without qualification. The words "which on no account one must spread abroad," stand in apposition rather than qualifying the kinds of information that are to be kept confidential. This is the reading in the World Medical Association's twentieth-century update of the Oath and in a minority of other interpretations.

This interpretation seems implausible on two counts. First, it is inconsistent with the dominant Hippocratic theme of always acting to benefit the patient. (It would prohibit disclosures in cases like Dr. Brown's, in which the physician believed disclosure would benefit the patient.) Second, as von Staden points out, the Oath is remarkably frugal in its use of words, "meticulously crafted and structured so as to avoid redundancy."[27] The nonrestrictive understanding of the reference of "things that ought not be spread abroad" would be unnecessary repetition. It would also prohibit the now-standard requirement of Tarasoff-like disclosures to warn third parties of serious threats. Either interpretation of the Oath's confidentiality provision is thus inconsistent with modern, secular medical morality and law. It is also inconsistent with the current American Medical Association and similar codes that authorize such third-party warnings.[28]

The Concluding Bargain

After the initiation oath and code of ethics, the Hippocratic Oath ends with a concluding bargain in which the physician acknowledges "if I fulfill this oath and do not violate it, may it be granted to me to enjoy life and art, being honored with fame among all men for all time to come; if I transgress it and swear falsely, may the opposite of all this be my lot."[29] The meaning of this concluding bargain is also open to various interpretations.[30] Although the hoped-for reward is expressed in terms of good reputation, it surely has a religious quality of providing for the physician's ultimate reward or punishment "for all time to come." In Christian theology, this is called the Pelagian heresy. It explicitly holds that the physician will get the reward of honor and fame for all time to come through his moral righteousness. It is justification by works, to use the theological terminology. The physician is to earn his salvation by faithfully keeping his pledge of morally right conduct with patients. If he fails, however, the opposite will be his lot.

If we examine the compatibility of the Hippocratic ethic with religious and secular ethics, we confront the stark challenge this reward/punishment ethic presents. There may be religious ethics that embrace this overt Pelagian deal, but orthodox Christianity would certainly find this troublesome.

The Metaethical Peculiarities of the Hippocratic Oath

The initiation section of the Hippocratic Oath ends with a promise that sounds very odd to modern ears—to share the precepts of the school with pupils who have signed the covenant and have taken an oath, "but to no one else." While modern medicine instills the norm that one of the central roles of a physician is to educate the patient about the basic notions of health and disease, this ancient cultic group actually swears not to provide such insights to laypeople. The patient is not to be trusted with the esoteric knowledge of the Hippocratic school. This special knowledge is potent and dangerous if it falls into the wrong hands.[31] Perhaps this is compatible with pre-Vatican II Catholicism when the mass was mystified by being spoken in Latin, but surely it is incompatible with Protestant notions that the layperson is capable of being trusted with the wisdom of the tradition as well as post–Vatican II Catholicism and modern secular notions of knowledge transmission.

The Oath appears to derive from a group that had many characteristics of a secret religious cult, which, if not Pythagorean, at least had many of the characteristics of a Greek mystery religion complete with severe restrictions on the dissemination of the secret knowledge of the sect.[32] As such, the epistemology of the Oath, the way the moral information is known and transmitted, is esoteric; it is not accessible to the uninitiated by natural, rational, or public means. Thus, we are in a position to contrast the Oath's moral epistemology with both secular philosophical moral systems and religious ethics that rely on natural theology as a source of moral knowledge.

Should there be any temptation to write off this injunction to secrecy as an ancient commitment abandoned by modern professional medicine, we shall see that, at least until very recently, modern professional medical organizations have continued to insist not only that they are the legitimate authorities on the content of the ethics of professional practice but that their moral knowledge was secret and not to be shared with laypeople. Professional groups vaguely in the Hippocratic tradition typically make one of two claims about why they can pronounce about the ethics of their members.

The Claim of a Professional Moral Ontology

Professional groups may claim that the group itself is the source of the norms, that it invents the norms and imposes the norms on its members. When in the 1970s the AMA was in the middle of a dispute about its position that it was unethical for its members to advertise, Russell Roth, the speaker of the AMA's House of Delegates, said that the profession "has imposed upon itself certain proscriptions which are often poorly understood by the public, such as the avoidance of any semblance of professional advertising, which is all right for almost everyone else expect physicians."[33] This claim seems to amount to the profession claiming that it, and only it, can know the norms for the profession because the professional group actually creates the norms. Of course, if they come up with the moral norms themselves, they are in a good position to claim expertise on their content. The idea that the professional group actually invents the norms and imposes them on themselves seems particularly naive, however. Almost no one really believes that groups of humans, even professional humans, generate moral norms out of whole cloth.

The absurdity of this claim is seen by noting that, if the professional group were literally the source of the moral norm, it would be logically impossible for someone to state that the professional group approves of a behavior, but it is nevertheless immoral. It would be impossible to say the professional group has an immoral position because, if the profession is the source of the moral duty and imposes that duty upon itself, its self-imposed obligations would be correct by definition. No one, not even members of the profession, if they are at all thoughtful, believes this to be true. Professional groups not only can but actually have made moral mistakes in their pronouncements from time to time.

The Claim of a Professional Epistemology

When pressed, a defender of professionally articulated ethics may concede that the norms come from some deeper, more ultimate source—from the deity, from the laws of nature, from reason, or some such ultimate origin. The defender of the profession's role in articulating norms for the profession may at this point claim that, even though the norms are ultimately grounded in some more ultimate source, the professional group has special expertise in knowing the norms, that knowledge about professional skills or experience in the profession is necessary to understand what is morally required of a member.

In the British euthanasia debate in 1970, Lord Brock, a member of the House of Lords as well as a physician, made the following claim: "As an ordinary citizen I must accept that the killing of the unwanted could be legalized by an act of Parliament, but as a doctor I must know that there are certain things which are part of the ethics of our profession that an Act of Parliament cannot justify or make acceptable."[34] Neither of these positions–that professional groups create their own norms or have the needed skills in knowing the norms—is defensible. There is nothing about being a member of a profession that gives one any special expertise in creating or knowing the moral norms for professional conduct. Being socialized into a profession certainly gives members specialized knowledge about the profession. In medicine, members of the profession certainly have unusually high levels of knowledge about medicine. Physicians know the Krebs cycle and other facts of physiology better than laypeople do. They may know better how to diagnose illness, what the possible treatments for an illness are, and what the patient's prognosis is. None of this implies, however, that they have expertise in knowing what conduct is morally appropriate—whether it is acceptable to tell a benevolent lie, kill for mercy, or prescribe a painkiller. In fact, all the knowledge in the world about the facts of medicine cannot give one a special expertise in making evaluative choices based on those facts. It cannot tell us whether it is better to refer a cancer patient to an aggressive oncology research center for the latest protocol or refer the patient to a hospice. It cannot tell us whether it is moral or immoral to perform an abortion on a pregnant woman. It cannot even tell us which among several drug therapies that will have some physiological effect is the right choice.[35]

Long ago I coined the term "generalization of expertise" to refer to the mistake of assuming that because a medical professional is an expert on the facts of medicine, he or she is also an expert on the value choices, including the moral choices, about medical practice.[36] That may still be my most significant contribution to the field of medical ethics. Occasionally, some member of a profession may have unusual expertise in articulating moral and other normative choices about conduct in a lay–professional relation, but, on average, there is no reason to assume that professionals are better than laypeople are at making these choices.

In fact, most members of any given profession are simultaneously members of other groups—religious, cultural, or philosophical—that also claim to have authority for knowing the general moral norms for human conduct and derivatively the special moral norms for practicing the various professions. Thus, a Roman Catholic physician should be expected to believe that morality is a matter of conforming to the natural moral law and that law is knowable by reason aided by church-mediated sources of revelation such as scripture, tradition, and church teachings. According to the committed Catholic physician, the people with recognized expertise in knowing the moral norms are the teachers of the church—the pope, church councils, and authoritative theologians such as Thomas Aquinas. Religious laypeople have a role as well, but that role is generally less authoritative. The Roman Catholic physician who is religiously a layperson who normally can claim no special expertise in moral theology is not one with high-order expertise in this hierarchy. Knowing all there is to know about medicine and the role of the physician does not place one in a position to claim special knowledge of the moral norms. If a serious Roman Catholic physician wanted to seek moral guidance and could choose between the chairman of the professional group's ethics committee who happened to hold moral views radically different from the Catholic church and a respected Catholic teacher of moral theology with expertise on medical morality, surely he would turn to the latter.

Likewise, I claim, any physician and any patient should turn for moral guidance to sources of moral knowledge that they respect. These would normally not be the ethics authorities of the profession or any other source within the profession.

The Hippocratic Ethic: A Bizarre Ethical Theory

Before considering the relation of the Hippocratic Oath to various religious and secular systems of medical ethics, we should note how unusual, how peculiar, indeed, how bizarre, the Hippocratic ethic is and how strange it would be for modern physicians to subscribe to it. More notably, we should recognize that it would be even more bizarre for modern patients to concur. Even if the Hippocratic Oath was appropriate for members of an ancient Greek cult, surely it is deficient for modern medicine. The central feature of the Oath is the Hippocratic physician's commitment to work for the benefit of the patient, but in most standard interpretations, this commitment prevails even when the patient does not agree and does not want the benefit the physician is offering. Patients may reasonably disagree that the physician's action would really benefit them.

In some cases, even if they concede that the physician's action would be beneficial to the patient, the patient may nevertheless not want the benefit. For example, physicians in the last stages of the Hippocratic era (roughly the 1960s and '70s) would sometimes perceive that heroic, last-ditch efforts to save a patient from an apparently terminal illness really were in the patient's interest, but nevertheless, the patient might want to decline these benefits. Patients might want to decline them because they disagree with the physician's judgment that the treatment would be a benefit, but they may also want to refuse the treatment even if they agree it would be in their interest. They may prefer to preserve their remaining family resources for the benefit of a spouse or children, for example. The Hippocratic ethic of benefiting the patient would not permit a physician to back off when patients wanted to decline a benefit in order to serve the interests of family members even though that surely is the morally right course.

The Hippocratic ethic is bizarre in embracing not merely Greek gods and goddesses but in viewing the craft of medicine as a closed community with privileged knowledge, knowledge that, by duty, should not be shared with those outside the cult. The ethical structure is odd. It claims that a physician (or medical student), by making a promise to his or her professional group, is thereby not only permitted but actually required to act in a particular manner to someone outside the group—a patient—even though the patient was never a party to the promising and may well object to the action the physician is taking. A fundamental flaw exists in an ethic that claims to generate duties by an act of promising when the promise is made not to the one toward whom one will be acting but rather toward some third party, in this case the professional group. It is even more odd when the group then claims that the lay population has no right to know the commitment that is made to the profession. Yet, as we shall see, the Hippocratic ethical tradition has continued, until very recently, to claim that its knowledge, including its moral knowledge, is private and not to be shared with outsiders.

The Hippocratic ethic is bizarre not only in its metaethical structure but also in its substantive, normative content. It is an ethic that, for archaic ritualistic reasons, prohibits surgery. It is an ethic that either restricts abortions that many believe are morally tolerable or, alternatively, restricts only those involving an archaic technique of the pessary. It is an ethic that holds out virtues of purity and holiness rather than the classic secular or theological virtues. It is an ethic that permits breaches of confidentiality for strictly paternalistic reasons even when the patient would not agree that disclosure would be beneficial. It is an ethic that would not permit disclosure of a credible threat of a patient to commit a homicide. It is an ethic that seems open to the charge that it involves a reward and punishment theory that is heretical. In the next chapter we trace the odd and chaotic history of the Hippocratic tradition, seeing how at many points in time physicians and laypeople have either felt compelled to modify the Hippocratic provisions or have simply ignored the Oath in favor of moral norms coming from other sources, usually religious or secular.

2

THE HIPPOCRATIC TRADITION

A Sporadic Retreat

ALTHOUGH THERE IS EVIDENCE of the Hippocratic school in ancient Greece (Hippocrates is mentioned in Plato), it was not the dominant Greek school of medical thought.[1] Others prevailed alongside it. Thus, when some follower of Hippocrates created an oath named in his honor, it is reasonable to assume the Oath applied, at most, only to one among many schools of medical practitioners. Kudlien emphasizes that the Oath is utterly unique even among Hippocratic writings. There was no hint of its acceptance in Greek or Roman medicine. He suggests it is even possible that it was written by a single, isolated physician with a peculiarly religious mind who was inspired to produce a literary document with religious and cult-like elements.[2] This raises the question of how the Hippocratic Oath rose to such prominence that it is often, if mistakenly, seen as the universal foundation for ethics in medical practice.

The Survival of the Hippocratic Tradition in Ancient and Medieval Culture

The first clear reference to the Oath occurs in the first century of the common era when Scribonius Largus refers to Hippocrates as "the founder of our profession" and then indicates that Hippocrates began his instruction with an oath.[3] Existing texts of Galen, a century later, never refer to the Oath.[4]

The evidence for the presence of the Hippocratic Oath in the medieval period is hard to come by. Carlos Galvao-Sobrinho says that references to the Hippocratic Oath are rare in late antiquity.[5] Antonio Garzya, analyzing medical ethics in the Byzantine Empire, makes reference to the Hippocratic corpus but no mention of the Hippocratic Oath.[6] He describes medical ethics of the Byzantine Empire as a hybridizing of Greek and Christian ethics. Jacques Jouanna notes that the Hippocratic Oath was not a major reference during the Byzantine period.[7] The Oath is not present in the known texts translated into Latin in the fifth and sixth centuries. Carol Mason Spicer and I, searching for references to the Hippocratic Oath in the Patristic church fathers, found only two references to the Oath in the first eight centuries of Christian history.[8] Both come from the fourth century, and both self-consciously distinguish Christian ethics for physicians from Hippocratic.

The first reference is found in Jerome's Letter LII:

It is your duty to visit the sick, to know the homes and children of ladies who are married, and to guard the secrets of noblemen. Make it your object, therefore, to keep your tongue chaste as well as your eyes. Never discuss a woman's figure nor let one house know what is going on in another. Hippocrates, before he will teach his pupils, makes them take an oath and compels them to swear fealty to him. He binds them over to silence, and prescribes for them their language, their gait, their dress, their manners. How much more reason have we to whom the medicine of the soul has been committed to love the houses of all Christians as our own homes.[9]

While Jerome speaks without hostility about the Hippocratic Oath, he clearly differentiates Christian "medicine of the soul" and reveals that Christians are not expected to swear such an oath.

The second reference, also in the fourth century, is in the writing of Gregory of Nazianzus, who refers to his younger brother, Caesarius of

Nazianzus, who held a number of court offices including that of physician. Gregory differentiates his brother from Hippocratic physicians:

"Among physicians he gained the foremost place with no great trouble, by merely exhibiting his capacity, or rather some slight specimen of his capacity, and was forthwith numbered among the friends of the Emperor, and enjoyed the highest honors. . . . By his modesty he so won the love of all that they entrusted their precious charges to his care, without requiring him to be sworn by Hippocrates, since the simplicity of Crates was nothing to his own."[10]

Once again, the Hippocratic Oath is recognized but clearly differentiated from Christian medicine, which is deemed superior. According to Galvao-Sobrinho, the only other instance of the Hippocratic Oath explicitly used as an oath prior to the eleventh century occurs in an anonymous treatise dated in the ninth or tenth century.[11] Called "Treatise J," it appears to have its origins in a northern European monastic center. The origins and use are unknown. This and other texts in the collection of the period reflect non-Christian and classical ideals in which the secular element predominated.[12] Treatise J contains a passing reference that implies that the physician takes the Hippocratic Oath: "Before the physician takes the Hippocratic Oath, and before he attempts surgery, he ought to heed words of wisdom."[13] Galvao-Sobrinho concludes that "it is impossible to know with certainty whether contemporary physicians really *took* the Hippocratic Oath or not."[14] Given the increasing influence of classical Greek culture by this time, it is entirely possible that the tension between Christian and Hippocratic ethics has been lost. Galvao-Sobrinho concludes this may well be more of a "bookish allusion to an ancient practice" than an actual contemporary practice. If this is the case, then the medieval status of the Oath is consistent with the pattern we see in modern times of physicians who are isolated from the substance of serious religious and philosophical scholarship, making uninformed reference to the Hippocratic Oath as a short-form placeholder for a serious ethical theory. Galvao-Sobrinho's conclusion is that the Hippocratic Oath "played a minor role in early medieval thought about medical ethics."[15] It reinforced ethical postures of the existing culture.

Especially, among those for whom subtle (and not so subtle) differences among ethical traditions passed over their heads, an occasional use of what was taken as the short-form summary of the classical Greek medical ethic provided rhetorical flourish. Even then, the Oath was used selectively. No use is made of the portions of the Oath dealing with the relation of masters and students or of the concluding reward/punishment bargain. As seen in Treatise J, overtly irrational sections, such as the prohibition on surgery, were ignored.[16] The Oath was well on its way to functioning not as a specific codification of norms of physician conduct but rather as a placeholder for the physician of good character, a useful symbol for commentators who are not philosophically or theologically sophisticated enough to grasp the tensions between the pagan cultic norms and those of the Christian or secular culture of the day.

The Oath Insofar as a Christian May Swear It

This pattern of assimilation of Christian and classical Greek culture continues in the later Middle Ages. The most significant challenge in the Middle Ages to one attempting to defend the thesis that the Hippocratic Oath is in critical conflict with various religious and secular systems of ethics comes from versions of the Oath that survive in a modified form, "In so far as a Christian May Swear It."[17] Beginning in the tenth century, manuscript references to the Hippocratic Oath appear in preserved manuscripts, although MacKinney describes the references as "second hand."[18] The earliest manuscript containing the actual text is from the thirteenth century.[19] Nevertheless, major surgery is required to make the Oath acceptable to the medieval Christian physician.

The most conspicuous document is a Christian version of the Oath that simultaneously reveals late medieval Christian acceptance of the Oath and a necessity to make significant changes in it. The text of "The Oath According to Hippocrates in so Far as a Christian May Swear It" is translated and analyzed by the editor of the Loeb edition of the Hippocratic works, W. H. S. Jones.[20] Three manuscripts of the Christian version are documented by Jones, referred to as the Urbinas, Ambrosianus, and Bononiensis manuscripts. Urbinas is the oldest, dating from the tenth or eleventh century. Ambrosianus is from the fourteenth century; Bononiensis, from the fifteenth.[21] The first two are written in the shape of a cross. Jones suggests that the Christian form was probably written some centuries earlier than the oldest of the three manuscripts, that is, before the tenth century.[22] He provides no support for this speculation, which strikes me as implausible given the almost complete absence of any surviving documentation of Christian interest in the pagan medical oath in the early Middle Ages. As we have seen, the only two references to it prior to about the ninth century both clearly differentiate Christian from Hippocratic medicine.

I am doubtful that the Christianized text traces back this far. Early Christians were acutely aware of the differences between Christianity and the pagan Greek religions. Both Jerome and Gregory, as we have seen, differentiate Christian medicine from Hippocratic and imply Christians do not take such an oath. There are no other surviving references to the Oath in the earlier centuries. It seems to me more reasonable that the attempt to Christianize the Oath must await the later Middle Ages when Catholic scholars were rediscovering classical thought. In the absence of any evidence of Christianized Hippocratic Oath-taking, I suspect the Oath "in so far as a Christian may swear it" dates from closer to the time of the existent manuscripts.

Still, we are left with the question of why Christians would want to take a version of a pagan Greek oath that is out of character for Christians in so many ways. Two hypotheses come to mind. First, it may be, as I have suggested, that by the beginning of the second millennium the time of the intense tensions between Christians and Greco-Roman beliefs was a distant memory. The rediscovery of the classical world, transmitted through Islamic scholarship to the doctors of the church, may have inclined Christian scholars, including Christian physicians, to absorb—for the time being—the pagan practice of oath-taking. Just as Aquinas could adapt Aristotle for Christian uses, so medical moralists may have cannibalized Hippocrates for Roman Christian purposes.

The second possibility is that the Christianized Hippocratic oaths may have been a product of physicians rather than theologians. Physicians rediscovering Hippocratic medicine with its commitment to effective strategies of secular explanation of disease and keen observation may also have encountered the Oath and chosen to adapt it for their purposes.

Regardless of why this occurred, the comparison of the original pagan text and the Christianized texts reveals that tensions remained between the two. A number of critical changes were needed to make a version acceptable to a Christian. The first and most obvious change was the deletion of the appeal to the Greek gods and goddesses. This was re-placed with an opening statement, "Blessed be God, the Father of our Lord Jesus Christ, who is blessed for ever and ever."[23]

Of more substance, the Christian form completely omits the entire first portion of the pagan oath, the portion that resembles an initiation ceremony and announces that the physician will regard his teacher as equal to his parents, provide money in time of the teacher's need, con-sider the teacher's offspring as equal to the student's own children, and provide the teacher's offspring with instruction without fee or indenture. Most critically, the language suggesting that the pagan oath treated knowledge as secret and potent—implying a setting of a Greek mystery religion—is abandoned. Absent is the suggestion that the precepts and instruction will be given only to those who have signed the covenant and have taken to the oath and to no others. The author of the Christian text felt compelled to omit all suggestions of a clan-like mystery cult or guild. Christianity, even in the late medieval period in which Greek culture was collapsed into the surviving Christian society, could not tolerate the implication of a pagan mystery religion.[24]

Turning to the second main section of the Oath, the ethical code, critical changes were incorporated into the Christianized version. The pagan prohibition on performing surgery is gone. If we are correct in suggesting that the objection to Hippocratic practice of surgery was con-cerned about ritual defilement with blood contamination, there is no place for this in a Christian code of physician conduct.

A change is also introduced into the abortion provision. While the pagan oath prohibited only the use of a pessary to produce abortion, the Christian revision is translated by Jones as "I will not give treatment to women to cause abortion, treatment neither from above or below."[25] Jones views this as a more definite and explicit promise. It is one that makes clear that all means of producing an abortion are unacceptable.

The final sentences of the pagan oath, which I refer to as a "concluding bargain," are also modified in the Christian version. Where the pagan Hippocratic physician hopes that he may keep the provisions of the oath on his own, thus gaining honor among all men for all time, the Christian physician makes clear that God must be the physician's guide and helper.[26]

What results is a late–Middle Ages assimilation of the pagan Hippocratic Oath now deemed characteristic of Greek culture with the Romanized Christian view of the world, what MacKinney has called "a fusion of classical antiquity with Christianity."[27] For this pre-Reformation moment, Athens and Jerusalem are less at odds.

We are left with no clear evidence to explain the late medieval appearance of explicitly Christian versions of the Oath of Hippocrates after about a millennium of either ignoring it or keeping it clearly differentiated from Christianity. The late–Middle Ages are, according to MacKinney, a period of secularization and "despiritualization" in medicine.[28] After centuries of monastic medicine, more secular and practical concerns are driving physicians at the time when Salernitan medicine emerges. MacKinney describes it as a period when "professional cleverness overshadows Hippocratic and Christian idealism."[29] Medical manuscripts of the time were often remarkably pragmatic and secular. One advised sending a messenger in advance to learn of the patient's condition so the physician will not appear ignorant. He is told to "pretend that the case is serious." This way, whether the patient survives or dies, the physician's reputation will be safe.[30] Thus it could be that physicians of the period attracted to the revised Hippocratic Oath were laypeople ignorant of the long history of tensions between pagan mystery religion and Christian theology. Alternatively, by this time, the differences between classical Greek thought and Christian views had receded so far into the background that even theologically trained scholars may have been attracted to the ancient classical statements and have set out to adapt them much as Aquinas and the scholastics did with Aristotelian thought. One way or another, we find in the late Middle Ages a rare moment in the history of medical ethics in which pagan Hippocratic and Christian ethics partially converged. Even then, however, the compilers of the Christianized version of the Oath felt compelled to make substantial omissions and revisions.

The Arabic Preservation of Hippocratic Ethics

The rediscovery of the Hippocratic Oath, as with the rediscovery of much of the classical Greek sources, occurs most importantly in the Arabic scholarship of the Middle Ages.[31] Even then, the presence of the Hippocratic text is sporadic. Many discussions of medical deontology do not mention it. For example, in the *Kamil as-sina'a al-tibbiya* by *'Ali ibn Al-'abbas al-Majusi*, an introductory chapter on medical deontology is based on the Hippocratic Oath, which is explicitly mentioned.[32] But in Constantine's translation (*Pantegni*, 1515) the reference to the Hippocratic Oath is omitted. Jacquart believes that this is because there were no Latin versions of the Oath before the fourteenth century, even though some elements of it and references to it can be found from the early Middle Ages on.[33]

According to Gotthard Strohmaier, the Hippocratic Oath had a more important role in medieval Islamic territories than in the Greek world.[34] Handbooks explaining the duties of the *muhtasib* (civil servant in charge of the public oversight of medical professions) contain the obligation of requesting the Hippocratic Oath of every physician exercising medicine in his district. The author retells the story of Hunayn, who relied on the Hippocratic Oath and his religion as an excuse for not giving a deadly poison to the Caliph. He cites a translation of the Hippocratic Oath in Ibn Abi Usaybi'a's *Muntahab siwan al-hikma* (which is also reproduced in Jones's *The Doctor's Oath*, 31–33). The translation is faithful to the original, except for the reference to Greek Gods. Bagher Larijani and Farzaneh Zahedi claim that the Hippocratic Oath was mandatory in Islamic hospitals in the tenth century.[35] They also mention a book by Haly Abbas inspired by Hippocrates but going beyond the Oath. But the author writes in a clearly monotheistic framework and insists on helping the poor.

Martin Levey sheds light on medical ethics in medieval Islam.[36] His *Medical Ethics of Medieval Islam with Special Reference to Al-Ruhawi's "Practical Ethics of the Physician"* contains an introductory essay on medical ethics in medieval Islam and a translation of al-Ruhawi's *Practical Ethics of the Physician* (*Adab al-Tabib*). The main focus of the introduction is the way Islamic religious ideas harmonized with Greek ethics. Greek rational ethics (Aristotelian virtue ethics) is seen as a means for man to attain oneness with God. The text itself contains references to Hippocratic ethics, but al-Ruhawi did not require the Hippocratic Oath since the profession was given only by God.

Iraqi scholar Joseph Habbi provides an account of the work of Hunayn ibn Ishaq (809/810–873), one of the most important translators of scientific and medical texts from the Greek. He translated the Hippocratic Oath into Syriac, and his nephew then translated it into Arabic.[37] Habbi also reviews three works on Islamic medicine by thirteenth-century writer Ibn Abi Usaybi'ah (1203–69).[38] One of them contains an oath called the 'Ahd or Qasam, which is similar to the Hippocratic Oath.

Arabic interest in Hippocrates also becomes reflected in the twelfth-century physician/rabbinical scholar Maimonides. He spent much of his life in Egypt and Morocco and wrote extensively on medical topics, including commentaries on a number of Hippocratic writings. These included a commentary on Hippocrates's aphorisms and several medical works attributed to Hippocrates. However, I can find no interest in the Hippocratic Oath.[39] In short, Arabic rediscovery of classical Greek texts creates a place for Hippocratic medical ethics in medieval Islam even though its presence is sporadic and is supplemented by uniquely Islamic influences.

Modern Hippocratic Ethics

In the modern period, the Hippocratic Oath has had moments of ascendency. Through long periods it lapsed into the status of a quaint, sometimes controversial relic that was often simply ignored.

Early Modern Medical Ethics

If we believe Sanford Larkey, sixteenth-century England relied on the Oath as a standard for medical moral conduct. However, he was writing in the 1930s and clearly had embraced the myth that the Oath is a timeless ideal of eternal prominence. He claims of the Oath that "in all ages it has been a guide to the physician in his relations to his patient and to society."[40] His naive premise is that the Oath for history "in all periods" was a model to the physician, a presumption that, as we have already seen, is surely incorrect. Not only did it fail to play this role in ancient Greece, it is virtually absent from all of the first millennium of Western history (not to mention many millennia of Eastern thought). Even Larkey's own analysis should give one pause. He identifies four independent English versions of the Oath in sixteenth-century England. The earliest existing text is from 1566, John Securis's *A Deterion and Querimonie of the Daly Enormities and Abuses Committed in Physick*. Others date from 1586, 1588, and 1597. The 1586 text is in Thomas Newton's *The Olde Mans Dietarie*, and the next is John Read's translation of Arcaeus, *A Most Excellent and Compendious Method of Curing Woundes*. Lastly, Larkey identifies Peter Lowe's *The Whole Course of Chirurgerie*, from 1597.

Already two-thirds of the century is absent from Larkey's analysis, even if we assume—without basis—that these texts represent a common recognition and acceptance of the Oath in the latter decades of the century. On the basis of these four texts, Larkey concludes that the Oath "reached a wide circle of medical readers."[41] Of course, there were Latin versions, which Larkey describes as being available as early as 1525. Still, none of this suggests that the Oath was widely influential in sixteenth-century England. My conclusion is that Larkey's primary sources reveal some degree of interest in the Oath in sixteenth-century England but that no evidence exists that the Oath was widely influential, much less that it was sworn by physicians upon graduation from their training.

It is even more difficult for me to assess the place of the Hippocratic Oath on the continent. The most thorough twentieth-century scholarship in English provides some clues. Winfried Schleiner, a professor of English from the University of California, Davis, with interests in Renaissance medical history, has produced a fascinating study titled *Medical Ethics in the Renaissance*.[42] He provides an extensive account of scores of sixteenth- and seventeenth-century physicians, primarily in southern Europe, who wrote on topics of the day in medical ethics. The issues included benevolent lying to patients as well as some fascinating, if arcane, problems in medical morality related to sexual issues—"removing seed" and syphilis. He is not addressing our issue of the place of the Hippocratic tradition in Renaissance medical ethics, but he provides considerable indirect evidence. The overall impression of his account of two hundred pages of perhaps sixty commentators in medical ethics is that there is precious little interest in the Hippocratic Oath or the moral tradition deriving from it.

As one might expect, many of the physician analysts of medical morality stand explicitly within the Roman Catholic tradition. They are engaged with the doctors of the Church, the papal authorities, and the moral agenda of these theologically inclined theorists. Some—for example Girolamo Bardi, who lived during the first two-thirds of the seventeenth century—studied under the Jesuits and obtained doctorates in both theology and medicine.[43] Reasonably enough, it really did not matter to them what Hippocrates or his followers (including the follower who crafted the Oath) might have thought about moral matters.

Similar absence of the use of Hippocratic ethics as authority occurred among the Jewish physicians that are prominent in Schleiner's account of Renaissance medicine in Europe. Elite Jewish physicians were exiled from Spain and Portugal as part of the edict that forced a migration of

Jews. Some became "new Christians," converts who, at least by public profession, abandoned their Jewish origins. For perhaps obvious reasons, many of these Jews and former Jews did not reference Talmudic sources for the medical ethical analysis. They often presented themselves as secular, rational physicians who were open to the use of Greek sources.

The exiled Portuguese Jewish physician whom Schleiner takes to be perhaps the most significant contributor to Renaissance medical ethics was Rodrigo de Castro. His *Medicus Politicus* incorporates passages from the Old Testament as well as secular "rational" analysis that relies on Greek sources. He emphasizes, however, that his sources are not selected because they are Greek, Arab, Hebrew, or Latin, but rather because "they speak the truth."[44] Thus it is striking that, when writing on medical ethics from this eclectic perspective, it is not Hippocrates that he cites but other classic sources. Commenting on the medical authors on which he relies, he says, "For they do not teach religion but medicine. Plato is my friend, as is also Socrates, but a closer friend is truth."[45]

To be sure, there are occasional references to Hippocratic medicine. The fascinating discussion of the medical problem called "suffocation of the mother" is oriented to the physician's moral dilemma brought about by the belief that hysteria in women was caused by an accumulation of something referred to as "female sperm," and that therapy included manual vaginal intervention sufficient to cause physical stimulation that would release the excess.[46] This therapy relied on ancient medical understanding of female physiology for which Hippocrates's understanding was sometimes cited.[47] Even when the ancient understanding of medical science was cited, however, it was often by reference to other figures, including Galen and Aristotle. Ian Maclean wrote, "The situation by the end of the sixteenth century is quite confused, but it may be said with a certain degree of confidence that the general context of medicine remains Galenist, while the work of Aristotle and the 'neoterici' is in dispute."[48] Hippocrates does not even make the list (except insofar as Hippocratic views were reflected in Galen).

Although there are occasional references to Hippocratic medicine to supplement the more frequent reference to Aristotle and Galen, the

striking observation for our purposes is that there is almost no citation of
the Hippocratic Oath. Even when Hippocratic sources are cited for ethical matters, it is for the most part not the Oath that is referenced but
writings believed to be Hippocratic, such as the *Epidemics* or letters mistakenly attributed to Hippocrates that had recently become available.[49]

There are complexities in this account of the marginal role of Hippocrates in Renaissance medicine, however. While Schleiner's book-length
account of the work of scores of physicians writing on medical ethics in
the sixteenth and seventeenth centuries gives only a very limited role for
Hippocrates and almost no role for the Oath, he mentions in passing the
existence of commentaries on the Oath.[50] In particular, he cites
Lutheran physician Johann Heinrich Meibom (1590–1655), who wrote
a commentary on the Oath. Meibom refers to the existence of seven
Renaissance commentaries on the Oath but goes on to acknowledge that
he has only been able to put his hands on two of them.[51] Thus the Oath
was not only available to Christian and Jewish physicians of the period
but it attracted some attention even if that attention was so slight that a
major figure could not locate the texts of commentaries.

Adding to the complexities of this picture is a remark of Jewish physician David de Pomis (1525–1600) in which, after supporting a point with
reference to the Oath, he adds parenthetically that all physicians subscribe to this Oath.[52] We are thus left with a picture that is as complicated as the Renaissance itself. In this time of the rediscovery of the
classics and openness to eclectic scholarship including Greek, Roman,
Arab, Jewish, and Christian sources, Hippocrates has risen to the level
of consciousness of the scholarly physician, and on rare occasion the
Oath attributed to him is incorporated into medical morality even if the
more normal and natural intellectual context is Jewish, Christian, or classic sources unassociated with the Hippocratic tradition.

The Eighteenth-Century Enlightenment

If Renaissance openness to the classics, including occasionally to Hippocratic authors, meant that Greek medicine was received with some

acceptance and Hippocratic ethics was at least not openly challenged, the eighteenth century presents a return to almost completely ignoring the Hippocratic Oath and related Hippocratic sources.

Since my contribution to the Gifford Lectures took place at the University of Edinburgh, it is appropriate to examine the impact of the Oath in the development of medical education at this institution. I researched this question in some depth during my stay as a fellow of the Institute for Advanced Studies in the Humanities in 1996 while I was working on the Scottish portion of my book *Disrupted Dialogue*. I was examining the dialogue between humanists and physicians in the English-speaking world. As part of that research I was permitted to examine the volumes of the university's "Laureation" book, an official register dating from the first university graduate in 1587 (more than a century before the existence of the medical faculty or even graduates in medicine) that contains the original signature of every graduate appended to a declaration called the "Sponsio Academica."[53]

Beginning with the first graduate—Robert Rollock, in 1587—every graduate has signed a sponsio. The signature has been attached to a short confession of faith or covenant. The wording was based on text first subscribed to by King James I and his household in 1581 and soon thereafter by "all persons of rank."[54] This text was incorporated into the Scottish National Covenant in 1638. By 1604, more than a century before the first medical degree was given by the university, professors as well as graduates were required to sign the oath, which included a pledge to remain affectionate and dutiful to the University of Edinburgh. Thus, its purpose was to affirm loyalty to the King, Scottish religion, and the university. A new version was adopted in 1639, but the function remained the articulation of patriotic, religious, and academic loyalty.

With the granting of the first medical degree in 1705, that graduate, David Cockburn, signed a sponsio that differed only slightly from the one signed by other students. It committed Dr. Cockburn to "maintain the Christian religion in truth and purity purged of all Popish errors."[55] The same document was signed by sixteen others who graduated with medical degrees before the establishment of the medical faculty in 1726 as well as by the two graduates from that faculty up until 1731. Thus, the origin of the oath-taking by medical graduates at the University of Edinburgh was a custom followed by all graduates of the university, a custom established more than a century before any medical degrees were granted. It had nothing to do with the Hippocratic Oath or any custom of medical student oath-taking.

A new version was adopted in 1731, but it still contained the Reformation Christian pledge and was in no way related to the Hippocratic Oath. That form was used until 1803, when a new form was adopted for medical students. It no longer contained the reference to the Christian religion or to "popish errors." The opening line now reads, "Whereas the distinction of a degree in Medicine is now to be conferred upon me, I solemnly promise before God, the Searcher of hearts, that I will to my latest breath abide steadfast in all due loyalty to the University of Edinburgh." It is in this version that we discover the first hint of a connection to the Hippocratic Oath. A single-sentence confidentiality provision is included that is closely related to the Hippocratic wording. The remainder of the text is still totally non-Hippocratic.[56] Thus, at the beginning of the nineteenth century the university's medical graduates are exposed to a Hippocratic sentence, but even then the core text and the tradition of oath-taking comes from the customs of the university and the broader society, and has no relation to medical education.

The thesis of *Disrupted Dialogue* is that medical ethics in the English-speaking world depends heavily on the quality of the dialogue between physicians and humanists. When that conversation is robust, as it was during the Scottish Enlightenment, the ethical content of medical ethical documents is dependent upon the debates in philosophical and religious ethics of the day rather than ancient professional medical sources.

John Gregory, the most significant figure of the Edinburgh development of eighteenth-century medical ethics, was in close communication with David Hume and other philosophical figures of the period—particularly his close relative, Thomas Reid, who was a major player in Scottish moral philosophy of the day.[57] Gregory, who taught philosophy at Aberdeen before evolving into a physician and professor of medicine, had a reasonably sophisticated knowledge of the major philosophical controversies in ethics of the day. He was, in fact, on personal terms with some of the great philosophical minds of the day. He had no interest in and no need for an ancient document such as the Hippocratic Oath.[58] It was philosophically naive and offered very thin content compared with the rich set of issues embedded in the philosophical subject matter of his own day and culture. Once a physician was significantly engaged with the contemporary ethical theories and issues of his day, why would he regress to a short, ancient, obscure, cultic code that failed to address matters of substance and failed to connect with the more vital philosophical theories of the time?

A similar claim can be made for the other major physicians contributing to medical ethics of the late eighteenth century. In England, physician Thomas Percival of Manchester was the dominant figure. His intervention into a local dispute involving the stress produced on health professionals by an epidemic resulted in the 1794 contribution titled *Medical Jurisprudence*. It was, in fact, a synthesis of contemporary thought on medical ethics. It was later revised and published as *Medical Ethics; or, a Code of Institutes and Precepts, adapted to the Professional Conduct of Physicians and Surgeons* and became the foundation of modern medical ethics for physicians in the English-speaking world.

Percival, educated in Edinburgh during the 1760s, was a product of the Scottish Enlightenment and quite well versed in the philosophical and theological controversies in ethics of the day. In addition to his *Medical Ethics*, he wrote other works in philosophy and morals.[59] He communicated with not only the utilitarian philosopher William Paley but also the anti-utilitarians Richard Price and Thomas Gisborne, and ended up carving out a subtle position incorporating some of both traditions.[60] As one deeply engaged in the philosophical discourse of the day, Percival had little use for or interest in the Hippocratic tradition.[61] His *Medical Ethics* reveals he has knowledge of the Oath but makes only passing mention of it—and then in a somewhat critical way. Percival is much more engaged in the social ethical issues of his day, as befits a physician schooled in the utilitarian and anti-utilitarian philosophers of the day and called into action by a controversy in an overworked public hospital in which the naive Hippocratic maxim of always working for the benefit of the patient would prove irrelevant—indeed, useless.

A similar story can be told in late-eighteenth-century America, where the leading medical figures such as Benjamin Rush, signer of the Declaration of Independence and mediator of the feud between John Adams and Thomas Jefferson, manifest similar Edinburgh enlightenment influence. Both Rush and Samuel Bard, the founder of Columbia's College of Physicians and Surgeons, were Edinburgh educated and critically engaged in the social and political debates of the day. Both wrote extensively in ethics but showed little interest in the Hippocratic tradition.[62]

As the eighteenth century drew to a close, so did the close communication between humanists and physicians, which left the elite physician leaders of the time engaged in the current philosophical debates that shaped their involvement in medical ethics. The result was that none of these enlightened physicians had much interest in the Hippocratic tradition in ethics. When they mentioned Hippocrates, it was in passing, often critical of the ethics, and usually citing the ancient Greek for his contributions to the development of empirical medicine rather than ethics.

The Rediscovery of Hippocrates in the Nineteenth Century

By the beginning of the nineteenth century, the era of the enlightened conversation between humanists and physicians was drawing to a close. The next generation of teachers at the medical school at Edinburgh was no match for Gregory and his colleagues. Gregory's son, James, who succeeded him as professor of medicine at Edinburgh, continued to write in philosophy, but he was rather unique and his contributions were minor. Most of James's colleagues at the medical school no longer had philosophical interests at all. They were absorbed by the explosion of scientific knowledge, the need to provide practical education for their students, and the imperative to compete with lesser medical schools for matriculants. A detailed inquiry in 1826 by the Commission for Visiting the

Universities and Colleges in Scotland provided a nine-hundred-page verbatim transcript of the opinions of the faculty on education including the medical school at Edinburgh.[63] The nearly unanimous view of the faculty was that time could not be afforded for education in philosophy, ethics, or other humanities subjects. It is in this relatively impoverished philosophical environment that physicians were left on their own in isolation to articulate the ethics of their profession.

The First American Professional Codes   In the United States, local medical professional groups began having to articulate ethics responses to various crises on their own. The first example arose in Boston in 1808. A code of ethics, referred to misleadingly as the "Code of Medical Police," addressed the norms of conduct for physicians.[64] This modest document, in comparison with the extensive works by Gregory and Percival, was a mere eleven pages and addressed primarily relations among practitioners. Topics include the norms for consultation, treating another physician's patients, care for colleagues and their families, quackery, and fees. Topics we would think of today as medical ethics—issues of consent, truth-telling to patients, euthanasia, abortion, and the like—were not addressed.

What is critical for our purposes is that the three leaders of the local medical society who were asked to write the document were respected senior surgeons—John Warren, Lemuel Hayward, and John Fleet. They had experience in medical education, medical editing, and leadership in the local medical society, but not in broader aspects of philosophy or the other humanities.[65] They had direct knowledge neither of contemporary ethics literature in the humanities nor of the older Hippocratic literature.

Warren, Hayward, and Fleet explain explicitly their method for producing what appears to be their only foray into medical ethics. They say they examined the works of Gregory, Percival, and Rush and "selected from them such articles, as seemed most applicable to the circumstances of the profession in this place."[66] In fact, virtually all the content of their brief document can be found in the second chapter of Thomas Percival's *Medical Ethics*, the chapter dealing with the relations of physicians among one another. No longer is there any engagement with the humanists of the day or their issues.

Still, in Boston, there is no evidence that physicians of early-nineteenth-century America made any use of the Hippocratic Oath. As I document at length in *Disrupted Dialogue*, similar stories can be told about the other state and local medical societies. New York produced a code in 1823 based primarily on Gregory and Percival. Only physicians are cited.[67] Baltimore and Washington produced codes in 1832 and 1833, respectively.[68] Both were relatively short and dealt primarily with intra-professional matters such as fees and included references to eighteenth-century predecessors in medical ethics.

The 1823 New York code is the first medical ethical writing of this period that briefly introduces the Hippocratic Oath. It references the Oath's pledge that medical students will provide support for their teacher in time of need.[69] Physicians writing about the ethics of their profession have lost contact with the discourse of the humanities of their time. They are forced to rely on commentators of previous generations, such as Gregory, Percival, and Rush. The nineteenth-century physicians writing these medical ethics codifications make reference to members of the previous generation of their own profession who were capable of knowing and understanding the philosophical controversies of their day, but the early-nineteenth-century physician-writers are themselves out of touch with the humanists who were articulating theoretical and practical concerns of their disciplines.

It is in this vacuum that the Hippocratic Oath begins to emerge. It offers a digestible, one-page moral summary that physicians can cite when they are no longer engaged in the more complex academic controversies of the day. Sometimes even the citation of the Oath is misleading. The developments in Philadelphia provide the most dramatic illustration.

Kappa Lambda and the Discovery of the Hippocratic Oath as a Symbol   The elite physicians of Philadelphia formed a mysterious, secret society reminiscent of the ancient secret Hippocratic cult.[70] Called the Kappa Lambda Society of Hippocrates, its attempt to emulate the original Hippocratic group is apparent. Potential members were elected to this fraternity-like club without being told they were proposed for membership. Election had to be unanimous. The new initiates were told that "the venerable Hippocrates of Cos may be considered as the remote founder of this Society."[71] At a formal initiation ceremony, new members swore an oath that was called the Hippocratic Oath. Like its Hippocratic predecessor, it was a secret oath. The initiation ceremony text tells initiates that the oath "you have just taken is in substance the same as was administered to the original Hippocratic physicians," but, bizarrely, the actual text had no resemblance to the classic Oath.[72] The oath administered to the nineteenth-century Hippocratic aspirants read:

OATH OR AFFIRMATION

You do [swear/affirm] that you will endeavor to exalt the character of the Medical profession by a life of virtue and honour—that you will keep the secrets, guard the reputations, and advance the interests of this Society and each of its members; and that you will never encourage any one to devote himself to the study of Medicine whose learning, talents, and honourable qualities are not such as to render him respectable in his profession, and worthy to be distinguished as a member of this Society.[73]

The Philadelphia pretender is written in the second person rather than the original Oath's first person. It contains none of the Hippocratic wording. It does not even address the core Hippocratic norm of working so as to benefit the patient. It really does not even concern itself with the profession of medicine. The focus is on the reputation and interests of the Kappa Lambda group.

It seems clear that the creators of this document could not have actually seen the Oath attributed to Hippocrates. They merely borrowed the name as an iconic symbol of a medical tradition that had something to do with ethics. Even though the organization often undertook activities more designed to promote the interests of physician-members such as setting a secret fee schedule that its members were allowed to charge for medical services, the members persisted in dressing this self-promotion conspiracy in the clothing of the revered ancient medical cult.

The group did undertake activities in the realm of ethics, but not Hippocratic ethics. It reprinted an abridged version of Thomas Percival's *Medical Ethics* and adopted Percival's "social compact" language, apparently not realizing how alien that would be to the style and concepts of the ancient Hippocratic cult.[74] Other chapters of Kappa Lambda existed in New York, Washington, Baltimore, and Lexington. They all embraced Hippocrates and the Oath symbolically associated with him. Hippocrates and his Oath were on their way back as symbols for the physician even if that physician had no real knowledge or understanding of the ancient tradition. Ethics for the medical profession had become isolated from broader philosophical and religious ethics, reduced to reprinting of British writing from decades past, which, no matter how philosophically astute in its time, was not the ethics of the nineteenth-century American period and was certainly not a manifestation of the true Hippocratic text.

Many Translations of Hippocrates in the Nineteenth Century

The nineteenth century was a time of resurgence of interest in the Hippocratic literature and especially the Oath. Some scholars in medicine actually returned to the Hippocratic texts. Editions of the complete Hippocratic writings began to appear with greater frequency, and often in the original Greek. Greek physician Adamantios Koraes produced an edition in 1792 while living in Holland and Amsterdam.[75] In the 1820s Karl Gottlob Kühn produced a twenty-six-volume edition of classical medical authors, including Hippocratic works. This edition included a Latin translation with critical and exegetical commentary. In 1834 Friedrich Reinhold Dietz, professor at Königsburg, produced a two-volume edition. The definitive Maximilian Paul Littré edition, which provided a French translation, appeared over two decades from 1839 until 1861.[76] In 1846 physician John Redman Coxe published *The Writings of Hippocrates and Galen Epitomised from the Original Latin*. Prior to this, on November 3, 1829, he had given a lecture clearly indicating his infatuation with Hippocrates as well as his sense that his hero had not been received well—"An Introductory Lecture in Vindication of Hippocrates Delivered in the University of Pennsylvania."

Works such as those by Coxe made some of the Hippocratic literature available in English or other modern languages, thus making them accessible to typical physicians or scholars not prepared in the classical languages. Coxe makes clear that the Hippocratic texts were not read by the typical physician of the day, even if he revered the so-called father of Western medicine. From the introductory section, "To the Reader," dated September 16, 1846, Coxe says:

> With the exception of a few of the Hippocratic treatises, an *English* translation has never appeared. Of the writings of Galen, not one has received that form, for the benefit of the English reader. And yet the names of both of these great men are familiar to our ears, as though they were the daily companions of our medical researches. Our teachers refer to them ex cathedra; our books continually quote them; and yet, not one in a hundred of the Profession, at least in America, have ever seen them, and if interrogated, could not inform us of what they treat.[77]

Meanwhile, in 1849 a linguistically able Scottish surgeon named Francis Adams produced an edition titled *The Genuine Works of Hippocrates translated from the Greek with a Preliminary Discourse and Annotations.* He also acknowledges "my author's works are very obscure."[78]

Thus, by the mid-nineteenth century, Hippocrates was beginning to claim a new status as a symbol of all that is noble in medicine and medical ethics, even if only a handful of scholars had ever examined the texts. Those scholars tended to be physicians with inclination toward classical studies who, no matter how learned in medicine and classical languages, were not in communication with the philosophical, theological, or moral arguments of the day. This meant that they were not aware of the potential conflicts between Hippocratic ethics and the major moral theories outside of medicine. Often, such as in the sophomoric Kappa Lambda society, physicians claimed they stood in the Hippocratic tradition and even claimed they were subscribing to the Hippocratic Oath when they had no knowledge of that ancient document and, in fact, produced a text suiting their own purposes that had no meaningful ties to the Hippocratic literature except its name.

The American Medical Association, 1847   One of the responses to the plethora of alternative medical options of the mid-nineteenth century was for proponents of rational medicine—what we now think of as orthodox, allopathic medicine—to come together to collectively ward off the challenges from their competitors. In 1847 American physicians gathered in Philadelphia to form the American Medical Association. Their first act was to form a committee to prepare a code of ethics. Sociologists of the professions tell us that a group such as physicians who want to establish their craft as having special status will claim authority to generate its own code of ethics, thereby conveying to the broader population that they are not mere business people out to promote their interests but are a collection of professionals, which means—by definition—a group committed to the welfare of clients. In the case of medicine, the physician's commitment is, supposedly, to benefit the patient. Although reaping secondary rewards of the profession, such as income and satisfaction, is an accepted part of being in a profession, the primary purpose is service to the patient—at least that is the image professional organizations want to project to the public. That stands behind the work of Isaac Hays and Jonathan Bell, the two leaders of the committee that wrote the original American Medical Association (AMA) code of ethics.[79]

That code shows very little connection to the Hippocratic Oath or the moral tradition derived from it. To be sure, the AMA's 1847 code shared with the Hippocratic core principle a commitment to benefiting the patient and protecting the patient from harm. There is, however, no evidence that Bell, Hays, or any of the members of the committee actively followed the Oath or even had serious knowledge of its content. The AMA committee's own document makes clear that the sources were the Anglo-American physicians of the late eighteenth century—Thomas Percival, John Gregory, and Philadelphia's own Scottish-trained elite physician, Benjamin Rush.[80]

It thus absorbed, perhaps unknowingly, the Scottish consequentialism of the Enlightenment. The great moral philosophers' unique view that morality requires choosing the course that will maximize good consequences—the view inherited from Adam Smith, Francis Hutcheson, and

David Hume, and brought into medical ethics by their physician-philosopher colleagues John Gregory and Thomas Percival—by the middle of the nineteenth century becomes the core of American professionally generated medical ethics.

There is not a word of Hippocratic text or reference to the classic Oath in the twenty-four-page 1847 AMA code. It is often perceived as compatible with the Hippocratic ethic, presumably primarily because of its consequence-oriented commitment. The major first section after an eleven-page introduction talks about the duties of physicians to their patients. They should work for the welfare of the sick, uniting "tenderness with firmness, and condescension with authority." The arrogant tone continues. The physician's mind "ought to be imbued with the greatness of his mission, and the responsibility he habitually incurs in its discharge." "Unnecessary visits [to the patient] are to be avoided, as they give useless anxiety to the patient, tend to diminish the authority of the physician, and render him liable to be suspected of interested motive."[81]

The next section addresses the all-important obligations of patients to their physicians: "The members of the medical profession, upon whom are enjoined the performance of so many important and arduous duties towards the community, and who are required to make so many sacrifices of comfort, ease, and health, for the welfare of those who avail themselves of their services, certainly have a right to expect and require, that their patient should entertain a just sense of the duties which they owe to their medical attendants."[82]

A list of obligations of patients is then enumerated:

1. Selecting a medical advisor who has received a regular professional education;
2. Preferring a physician whose habits of life are regular;
3. Faithfully and unreservedly communicating to their physician the supposed cause of their disease;
4. Never wearying his physician with a tedious detail of events or matters not appertaining to his disease;

5. Obeying the prescriptions of the physician promptly and implicitly;

6. Avoiding, if possible, even the friendly visits of a physician who is not attending him;

7. When a patient wishes to dismiss his physician, declaring his reasons for so doing;

8. Sending, when practicable, for the physician in the morning, before his usual hour of going out; and

9. After the patient's recovery, entertaining a just and enduring sense of the value of the services rendered him by his physician (for these are of such a character that no mere pecuniary acknowledgment can repay or cancel them).[83]

Two additional chapters of the AMA document push beyond the Hippocratic principle's limited focus on what the physician owes the patient. In chapter 2 the AMA adds a serious discussion of what physicians owe to each other.

The real difference comes in chapter 3, the chapter devoted to duties of physicians to the public and the obligation of the public to physicians. I suggest three major problems with the Hippocratic ethic: its individualism, its consequentialism, and its paternalism. The AMA in 1847 remains totally consequentialistic; it says nothing of any human rights, any duties based on natural law or other deontological theories such as those related to Kantianism. It remains paternalistic. The key movement away from Hippocratic ethics for the AMA is a buy into a set of social ethical commitments—to require the physician to serve the society and to expect that society owe him or her something. To be sure, these socially directed concerns are subordinated to the traditional focus on the benefits for the individual patient, but the nineteenth-century discovery of concern about public health and the Enlightenment extension of consequentialism to the welfare of the community was important for professionally generated medical ethics. We saw it in a modest way in Percival, who was contending with the moral chaos of an epidemic. It appears more explicitly in the AMA in 1947 and is a significant departure from the Hippocratic perspective.

The AMA of the mid-nineteenth century holds that "it is the duty of physicians to be ever vigilant for the welfare of the community."[84] It notes specifically matters of "public hygiene." It even endorses a legitimate role for physicians in coroners' inquests, an area where the patient's interest can easily conflict with that of society. It acknowledges the physician's duty to respond to cases of patient poverty but quickly moves to protect the financial interests of its members by pointing out the need for "pecuniary acknowledgment" for public services in areas such as certifying the inability of persons to perform public service for the military or jury duty. The opening of organized medicine to duties to benefit the public is an important innovation in professional ethics. It points to the existence of significant differences within professionally generated ethics.

What has not changed from the Hippocratic tradition is the AMA's continuing normative commitments to consequentialism and paternalism. In addition, the AMA retains the traditional Hippocratic metaethic in which the professional group generates the code of ethics with no participation of medical laypersons. The AMA differs from the Hippocratic Oath in not insisting that its ethic is secret. The AMA did not claim that laypeople could not understand the AMA's ethical pronouncements, and it did make its positions available to the public.

By the 1840s American medicine was fragmented, with several schools or styles of practice competing for customers. Attempting to establish a unique moral legitimacy for allopathic medicine is generally recognized as the function of the AMA's code. What we would think of as orthodox allopathic medicine was battling with alternatives, including homeopathy, hydropathy, Grahamism, physiomedicalism, and Thomsonianism, which relied heavily on natural botanicals. It also had to contend with faith healers and all manner of charlatans. Many of these alternatives involved more conservative approaches, evidence of some reaction to harsh interventions of earlier decades such as the use of bloodletting and mercury compounds.

Primum non nocere: A Non-Hippocratic Alternative It is perhaps in this context that a popular slogan routinely confused with the Hippocratic Oath's core commitment was first introduced. If physicians or laypeople are asked to summarize the Hippocratic Oath, they will often reply with a stock maxim, "primum non nocere"—"First of all, do no harm." A number of contemporary books use the phrase.[85] I have a thick file of physician articles and letters to medical journals that spout the phrase, assuming it is Hippocratic and assuming the phrase settles the particular moral issue they are addressing.

The fact that the slogan is in Latin should give one pause. In fact, the phrase is not found in the Hippocratic Oath or any other Hippocratic writing. The Oath's key commitment is to have the physician benefit the patient according to his ability and judgment as well as protect the patient from harm. In current philosophical parlance it commits to beneficence as well as nonmaleficence—benefiting as well as protecting from harm. In the Oath, the two are given equal weight. Certainly, there is no "first of all" attached to the nonmaleficence principle. The Hippocratic slogan also adds a uniquely paternalistic twist to beneficence by specifying that the benefit is to be according to the physician's judgment.

Some have tried to associate the "primum" slogan with a passage in the Hippocratic writing, *Epidemics*, where the author says, "As to diseases make a habit of two things—to help or to do no harm." Still, this is a simultaneous and balanced commitment to beneficence and nonmaleficence. No hint of "primum" appears in the text.

Several of us sought for years to find the slogan's origins without success.[86] Jonsen offers several interpretations, some of which simply remove the "primum," that is, the "first of all" priority on not harming so that "primum non nocere" is remolded into the classic Hippocratic formula. That and Jonsen's other interpretations all fail to give adequate attention to the slogan's conspicuous "first of all" term.

For many years I suspected that the likely true meaning of the phrase was most easily understood in the context of mid-nineteenth-century medical conflicts between allopathic physicians and the more conservative, naturalistic competitors who believed that the body will heal itself if humans stay out of the way and let nature take its course. They opposed harsh, potentially dangerous interventions such as the use of mercury. They insisted that the moral priority was to first make sure the intervention would not do harm before considering whether it might do good. In current philosophical jargon, nonmaleficence was "lexically prior" to beneficence; it had to be satisfied before one turned attention to producing benefit. It was a moral maxim that gave a rank ordering to nonmaleficence over beneficence. Nonmaleficence must be satisfied before one takes up pursuit of benefit.

Recently, strong support has appeared for this hypothesis that "primum non nocere" had nineteenth-century origins related to the movement toward more conservative treatment strategies. Cedric Smith published an essay in 2005 titled "Origin and Uses of *Primum non nocere*—Above All, Do No Harm!" Independent of the searching that I and others have done to find the roots of the primum slogan, he analyzed a vast literature rejecting suggestions that it comes from Hippocrates, Galen, or the sixteenth-century author Ambroise Paré, all of which fail to provide the source. Smith finds the first occurrence of it in an essay of English physician Thomas Inman in 1860.[87] Smith goes on to show that Inman thought he was quoting the famous seventeenth-century physician Thomas Sydenham, but Smith shows that, in fact, the phrase is nowhere to be found in any of Sydenham's extensive writing. It appears that Inman was so embedded in the medical conservatism of the mid-nineteenth century that he felt comfortable attributing to his famous predecessor the insight of giving priority to not harming.

This conservative ethic is then at odds with the Hippocratic ethic that treats beneficence and nonmaleficence as co-equals to be satisfied by some integration of the positive and negative effects of an intervention. In this one respect the Hippocratic ethic is like Benthamite utilitarianism. The positives are to be noted for each alternative therapy under consideration, and the negatives are to be subtracted so that the physician pursues what he (always masculine, at least in classical Hippocratic ethics) judges will maximize the patient's expected net benefit.

In other versions of the Hippocratic benefit/harm calculation, the benefits are compared with the harms by calculating their ratio. The treatment option with the greatest ratio of benefit to harm is preferred. These
two methods of comparing benefits with harms (subtracting harms or
calculating their ratio) can produce different moral imperatives in certain
cases. Sometimes the treatment that has the best ratio of benefit to harm
may also produce a smaller difference if one subtracts expected harms
from expected benefits. In other words, even if one remains committed
to the traditional Hippocratic imperative of benefiting the patient and
protecting the patient from harm, there is not a single, unique set of
behaviors required. Different Hippocratic physicians, each committed to
following the Oath faithfully, can feel required to choose different therapies because they choose different strategies for comparing benefits and
harms. The fact that even an orthodox, classical Hippocratic physician
can calculate benefits and harms in more than one way is a part of my
reasons for claiming in *Patient, Heal Thyself* that physicians cannot be
expected to determine definitively what will benefit patients.[88]

What is not called for by the Hippocratic ethic is a rank ordering of
nonmaleficence over beneficence. There is no justification for doing no
harm "first of all." The "primum non nocere" slogan, taken literally, which
requires that physicians give first priority to making sure they never hurt
a patient with their actions, is an ultraconservative maxim. It could be
satisfied completely if the physician never did anything for any patient.
That would fail to do important goods, but it would always avoid actively
doing harm. While nineteenth-century physicians did not literally follow
the rule to its logical conclusion of doing nothing, they felt pressured to
act cautiously, a mandate not explicitly called for by the original Oath.
Thus, by the middle of the nineteenth century, professionally generated
codes of ethics that focused on benefiting the patient and protecting the
patient from harm were beginning to show significant variation from the
classical Hippocratic maxim. Some proponents calculated net benefits
by subtracting in Benthamite fashion the harms from the benefits; some
calculated ratios of benefit to harm. Still others insisted on focusing first
on not harming, and only after that requirement was satisfied was effort

to benefit the patient undertaken. From the time of Percival under the influence of Scottish consequentialism, doors were beginning to open to consideration of benefits to the public as well as the patient. The AMA of 1847 opened this non-Hippocratic door still further. Still, professionally generated medical ethics was isolated from the alternative sources of ethics for patients and health professionals—the religious and secular philosophical traditions. There was no reference to human rights—either the rights of patients or the rights of physicians. There was no Kantian notion of moral duty independent of what produced good consequences. There was no natural law, no Talmudic notion of covenantal law, no Catholic notion of papal or Church council authority, no Protestant notion of the layperson as interpreter of scripture.

Hippocratism and Its Professional Alternatives in the Twentieth Century

Revisions of the AMA Code   Since the initial generation of the AMA Code of Ethics in 1847, many revisions have occurred. The most significant appeared in 1903, 1912, 1947, 1957, 1980, and 2001.[89] That the AMA by now sees itself as standing in the tradition of the Hippocratic Oath is made clear in the initial pages of the current AMA Code, which starts with reference to the Oath and describes it as having "remained in Western Civilization as an expression of ideal conduct for the physician." In fact, we have seen that the original AMA Code was not derived from the Hippocratic Oath and seems more or less oblivious to it. The subsequent changes in the AMA Code do not rely in any significant way on the actual Oath.

The original tension between the allopathic practitioners who were members of the AMA and the competing systems of practice waxed and waned. At times the AMA saw fit to impose strict prohibitions on cooperation with practitioners from other schools of medicine. At other times this tension lessened and legal concerns led to a reduction in efforts to prohibit cooperation.

By 1957 a change of format led to a redrafting of the Principles of Medical Ethics so that the ideals were presented in a short, one-page list of ten principles.[90] The overall normative content, however, does not differ substantially from the 1847 document. There was still an emphasis on benefiting the patient. There was perhaps a heightened recognition that physicians have duties to the public as well as the individual patient. At least four of the ten principles explicitly acknowledge duties to the public: to determine the propriety of physician conduct in relation to the public (from principle 1); to safeguard the public against physicians deficient in character (principle 4); to breach confidentiality if necessary to protect the welfare of the community (principle 9); and, most importantly, to improve the health and well-being of the community (principle 10).

The 1957 codification retains many of the concerns that could be seen as self-serving: to avoid associating with anyone who fails to follow methods of scientific healing (presumably, such as mesmerists and faith healers as well as charlatans). The physician may choose whom he will serve. There are provisions governing the ever-sensitive matter of professional fees and charging for selling remedies to patients.

Not present in the 1957 principles was any evidence of historical, conceptual, or linguistic links to the Hippocratic Oath. Equally obvious was the complete absence of any hint of the moral perspective of rights or deontological duties. There remained a medical paternalism seen, for example, in the provision that the physician may disclose confidential information when necessary to protect the patient. There was no consideration that moral norms for physicians might have their grounding outside the profession, in the religious or secular moralities of the surrounding culture. No layperson was given any opportunity to contribute to the discussion of the norms for professional conduct or even the norms for lay–professional relations. The authority for adjudicating disputes about physician conduct rested entirely within the profession in the hands of a committee made up entirely of physicians.

It is not until the revision of 1980 that cracks begin to appear in this professional facade. At that point the society was well into a cultural revolution that was influenced by the major rights movements of the previous two decades. There had been an active antiwar movement and movements for civil rights, women's rights, and student rights. The language of liberal political philosophy and, in the United States, the founding fathers, had become dominant.

James Todd, a key figure in the mid-1970s case of Karen Quinlan, had emerged as a major player in the AMA and was appointed to chair a committee to look at the revision of the AMA's Code of Ethics.[91] The product, approved at the AMA House of Delegates meeting in 1980, was a major change in the AMA's ethics.

The new Code, adopted in 1980 and published in 1981, contained for the first time in any ethics document produced by a professional medical organization the language of rights. ("A physician shall respect the rights of patients, colleagues, and other health professionals, and shall safeguard patient confidences and privacy within the constraints of the law."[92]) Gone was the paternalistic authorization to breach confidences when it was perceived by the physician to be in the patient's interest to do so. On the other hand, the qualification that confidences should be preserved "within the constraints of the law" was an acknowledgment that American law had just determined that health professionals had a duty to break confidences to protect third parties from credible threats of grave bodily harm.[93]

The report of the Todd committee contained a remarkable acknowledgment of a metaethical change. The report began by stating that the "intent of the revision was to clarify and update the language, to reach a proper stance between professional principles and contemporary society and to eliminate any reference to gender." It went on to comment on a major shift in the metaethics: "The profession does not exist for itself, it exists for a purpose, and increasingly that purpose will be defined by society."[94]

This was reflected in the recognition that the broader society had a role in deciding the limits of confidentiality when the patient's behavior could be of danger to others. It would determine the moral limits on physician advertising. It would articulate the norms for the patient's rights (such as the right to consent or refuse medical treatment). The 1980 change was the watershed in the abandonment of patient-benefit ethics in favor of a more rights-oriented ethic and the abandonment of the exclusive authority of the profession in determining the moral norms for the health professional and the patient.

The British Medical Association   Similar evolution was occurring in organized professional medicine in Britain. Since the time of Percival, British professional medical ethics had not made extensive progress. The British Medical Association (BMA) considered writing a code of ethics in the 1850s but never completed its work.[95] No further evidence of ethics activity of the BMA appears until the mid-twentieth century. By 1963 the *Member's Handbook* contained a chapter on medical ethics. In 1970 the case of British physician Dr. Brown, described in chapter 1 of this volume, led to revising the BMA's confidentiality provision. Dr. Brown was accused of breaching the confidentiality of an adolescent patient by telling her father that she was taking birth control medication. Tried before the General Medical Council, Brown was acquitted of all charges on the grounds that the Hippocratic Oath, the British Medical Association, and the American Medical Association all recognized the duty of the physician to protect the well-being of the patient.[96] Soon after the decision the BMA Ethical Committee recommended a revision of its code of ethics to remove the paternalistic exception clause to its confidentiality provision.[97] The British were on their way to abandoning the more paternalistic position, a move that the American association took until 1980 to complete.

The World Medical Association Declaration of Geneva   During this period, the world of medicine was undergoing dramatic changes. It had been jolted by the outrageous and embarrassing participation of German elite physicians in the medical research and extermination programs of the National Socialists.[98] There is ample evidence that the "medical ethic" deviated radically from more traditional ethics that simply committed the physician to benefit the individual patient. National Socialist medical ethics embraced some elements of Hippocratic medicine and rejected Jewish and Christian ethical principles.[99] It is clear that the world of professional medicine had to respond aggressively following the war to assure the public that physicians were, in fact, still committed to working for the welfare of the patient.

The World Medical Association (WMA), the consortium of national professional medical organizations, responded by adopting in 1948 what it called the Declaration of Geneva.[100] Remarkably, the WMA explicitly embraced for the first time a somewhat updated paraphrase of the original Hippocratic Oath. The key sentence stated, "The health of my patient will be my first consideration." It was the WMA's way of reaffirming the duty of the physician to remain loyal to the patient's welfare and to forcefully renounce any tendency of the profession to desert the patient in favor of broader societal projects. While the AMA was moving toward a more responsible balance of societal interests in public health, medical research, and other public goods, the WMA was retreating to Hippocratism.

The WMA Declaration of Helsinki, 1962   The WMA's retreat to Hippocratism would soon begin to pose problems for the association. In particular, people began to realize that if WMA physicians worked for the health of their patient, societal concerns such as research designed to produce generalizable scientific knowledge took a back seat. In 1962 the WMA adopted the Declaration of Helsinki, a code addressing ethical issues of human subject research. That code was revised in 1964 and several times since then. The core idea was that the WMA acknowledged that, in a world in which medicine relied on systematic scientific research, sometimes a physician had to engage in behaviors involving patients that were not designed specifically for the benefit of the patient. Thus, the WMA's Declaration of Helsinki endorsed research it called "nontherapeutic," that is, research unconnected with therapeutic intent. Even in the case of the treatment of patients, research combined with patient care would necessarily involve procedures undertaken for the purpose of producing knowledge rather than benefiting the patient. In both cases, the WMA introduced a concept new to professionally generated codes of ethics—the notion of "free consent" after the patient or subject has been informed. In the case of research combined with professional care, this consent should be obtained "if at all possible." In the case of so-called nontherapeutic research, consent should be obtained unless the subject is incompetent, in which case the consent of the legal guardian should be obtained. Thus, by the 1960s the WMA had opened the door to physician behavior that deviated from Hippocratic standards of patient benefit, although in clinical medicine unconnected with research it retained its Declaration of Geneva, its updated Hippocratic paraphrase.

The Nuremberg Code   The scurrying of professional associations following World War II to adopt positions that would repudiate the National Socialist collaboration of physicians was stimulated in part by an important nonprofessional event immediately following the war—the Nuremberg trials. While the international professional association of physicians, the World Medical Association, was vigorously reaffirming its Hippocratic, patient-benefiting commitment by adopting the Hippocratic Oath paraphrase, the Declaration of Geneva, the world lay community was undertaking a major event in international law that led to the trial, conviction, and in some cases execution of Nazi war criminals, including some Nazi physicians. This would set the stage for the radical change in the WMA leading to the Declaration of Helsinki.

One of the most important and lasting products of that trial was a code of ethics for the conduct of medical research involving human subjects. Called the Nuremberg Code, it set out an international standard for the ethics of such research.[101] The international community and its agents at the trials faced a momentous choice that led to a different stance than the one originally adopted by the medical professional organization. It had two options if it was to establish a firm moral standard to protect subjects of research so that the Nazi atrocities could never again be tolerated.

One option, the one chosen by the WMA when it adopted its Declaration of Geneva, would have been to affirm the moral principle of the Hippocratic Oath—that physicians should always work for the benefit of patients and protect them from harm. That surely would have meant the prohibition of the Nazi research. The problem was that, logically, it would also have prohibited even the most benign, useful, and important studies as well. Medical research is distinguished from clinical therapy by the intention of the actors. Medical research by definition involves interventions undertaken to produce generalizable knowledge, not for the immediate benefit of the person upon whom the experiment is conducted. The Hippocratic principle of always working for the benefit of the patient would prohibit in principle all such research activities. Interventions on normal subjects who are not ill most obviously could not be undertaken by physicians holding to the Hippocratic principle. Even research on ill people could not proceed. Efforts to try out some novel or innovative therapy for a patient whose medical condition is not successfully treated with standard therapies could continue, but that is not what we mean by research. The gold standard strategies for research—randomization, blinding of both investigator and subject, controlling of variables and the like—are not for the purpose of benefiting the patient; they are for the purpose of producing generalizable knowledge. All procedures and techniques undertaken to produce knowledge rather than to help a patient would be excluded under the Hippocratic standard.

The contributors to the Nuremberg trials realized that reaffirming the Hippocratic principle for all future physician behavior—including research activity—would necessarily bring even the most innocent research to a halt. Instead, they adopted a set of ten principles, the first two of which are the most critical. The second principle holds: "The experiment should be such as to yield fruitful results for the good of society unprocurable by other methods or means of study, and not random and unnecessary in nature."[102]

Standing by itself, this is a repudiation of the professional Hippocratic standard because it explicitly affirms physician conduct for the good of society even if it is not for the benefit of the patient. In fact, such conduct is consistent with efforts that are likely to cause harm to patients. In order to prevent the abuses of the Nazi research, the authors of the Nuremberg Code inserted another principle and gave it the position of first place in the code: "The voluntary consent of the human subject is absolutely essential. This means that the person involved should have legal capacity to give consent; should be so situated as to be able to exercise free power of choice, without the intervention of any element of force, fraud, deceit, duress, over-reaching, or other ulterior form of constraint or coercion; and should have sufficient knowledge and comprehension of the elements of the subject matter involved as to enable him to make an understanding and enlightened decision."[103]

With this remarkable provision, the international community overturned a millennia of professionally generated ethics for physicians and established a standard grounded not in esoteric professionally controlled morality but in the rich history of liberal political philosophy and international law. This provision not only endorsed physician conduct not designed to benefit the patient and protect the patient from harm; it also endorsed a radically different source of authority for medical morality—the philosophical traditions independent of professional hegemony. Adopting the Nuremberg Code made clear, as never before, that laypeople as well as those who happened to be medical professionals had other sources to which they could turn—sources grounded in religion and philosophy—for establishing an ethic for lay–professional relations in health care. In the remainder of this book I pursue the central purpose of my contribution to the Gifford Lectures: I examine more closely these other sources of medical morality and how they sometimes conflict with professional sources when it comes to the grounding of ethics and the authority for knowing its content as well as the substantive norms themselves.

The first and most conspicuous place that these professionally generated sources might come into tension with other sources is in the activities of medical schools related to their socialization of medical students into the ethical tradition they attempt to instill in the students. The next chapter looks at the cacophony of professional, religious, and secular instruction in ethics transmitted to medical students in various medical schools. Following that, I examine the possibility of grounding professional ethics in theological systems of belief and more secular philosophical systems.

3

THE CACOPHONY OF CODES IN MEDICAL SCHOOLS AND PROFESSIONAL ASSOCIATIONS

O NE POINT OF CONTACT between the physician and various professional codes (the Hippocratic and its alternatives) is in the ritual of oath taking that occurs in medical schools. Long part of the stereotype of medical education, the image of graduating medical students standing, raising their right hands, and reciting in unison some professionally generated oath is fixed in the public consciousness.

Problems with Medical School Oath Taking

While oath taking is part of the lore of our understanding of the crowning moment in medical education, the actual practice is more complicated than the image would suggest and it raises some very difficult moral issues. For example, why should a group of young people, usually fresh out of college, suddenly surrender the moral traditions they have learned from their families and through their churches or secular philosophical equivalents, and unanimously pledge to conduct the rest of their professional lives according to some specific code, Hippocratic or otherwise? It is absurd to think that four years of medical school should convert entire classes from their basic moral systems to one that they would suddenly come to adopt. More absurdly, as we shall see, different schools offer different oaths and pledges for their students in spite of the fact that the graduates will soon be moving on to hospitals or medical practices they share with graduates of other schools that have extracted a different oath or pledge from their students. Moreover, they will practice medicine on patients who cannot be expected to share in the ethical stance incorporated in the texts that schools have inflicted on their students.

The Sporadic History of Oath Taking

We have already seen that the practice of oath taking at the most important Scottish medical school had, in its origins, nothing to do with medical education. The *sponsio* was a pledge required of all graduates (and all faculty). Those who took the pledge promised loyalty to the university, the king, and the Scottish Covenant. When medical degrees were added to the university agenda many years after the beginning of the practice, medical students were also required to take the same oath. In the rest of the eighteenth century in Scotland and England there was little interest in the Hippocratic ethic. In the United States, city and state medical societies did not endorse or even know much about the Oath. The one group that made specific reference to an oath by that name was, in fact, referring to an entirely different text. The AMA's founding led to a code of ethics, but it was not linked to the Hippocratic Oath.

Oath Taking, 1928

We have data from throughout the twentieth century about oath taking at medical schools in North America. The patterns are quite revealing and troubling. Schools have been surveyed several times beginning in

1928. At that time only eighteen of seventy-four schools that responded used an oath. Only five of these were the unmodified Hippocratic Oath (see table 3.1). Five others used something identified as a "modified Hippocratic Oath." Eight others used some other oath. That leaves fifty-six that did not use an oath at all.

Oath Taking, 1958

By 1958 oaths were much more widely used—sixty-nine of ninety-six schools that responded to the survey used an oath, but only seven still used the unmodified Hippocratic document (see table 3.2). Fourteen others used what was termed a "modernized" version of the Oath, but most used some other text—the Declaration of Geneva or some other document.

Oath Taking, 1977

The next survey was in 1977, at which time 6 of 128 schools used the unmodified Hippocratic text and 45 others used a modified version. Still, the majority used some other document (the Declaration of Geneva

Table 3.1   Use of Oaths in North American Medical Schools, 1928

	Medical Schools in United States and Canada	
	Number	*%*
Used an oath	18	24.8
No oath	56	75.6
TOTAL	74	100
Classical Hippocratic Oath	5	
Modified Hippocratic Oath	5	
TOTAL use of Hippocratic Oath	10	55.6
Other oath	8	44.4
TOTAL	18	100

Source: Carey, "Formal Use of the Hippocratic Oath."

Table 3.2   Use of Oaths in North American Medical Schools, 1958

	Medical Schools in United States and Canada	
	Number	%
Used an oath	69	72
No oath	27	28
TOTAL	96	100
Hippocratic Oath	7	10.1
Modernized Hippocratic Oath	14	20.3
Declaration of Geneva	12	17.4
Other	32	46.4
Various	3	4.3
Undesignated	1	1.5
TOTAL	69	100

Source: Irish and McMurry, "Professional Oaths and American Medical Colleges."
Note: Medical schools in the United States = 84; medical schools in Canada = 12.

or the Prayer of Maimonides, for example) or used nothing at all (see table 3.3).

Oath Taking, 1993

By 1993 almost all North American schools were using an oath, but only one out of the 150 schools surveyed remained loyal to the unmodified Hippocratic Oath (see table 3.4). Another 67 used what was termed a modified or modern Hippocratic Oath, but a majority used some other oath, such as the Declaration of Geneva, the Prayer of Maimonides, or the newer oaths attributed to Luis Lasagna, the Osteopathic Oath, or some other text. The single school using the unmodified oath was the State University of New York at Syracuse. I have been informed that that school no longer uses it.

Thus, never in the twentieth century has a majority of schools in North America used the Hippocratic Oath, even in some modified form. Almost all schools have seen fit to at least make some changes, and the

Table 3.3   Use of Oaths in North American Medical Schools, 1977

	Medical Schools in the United States and Canada	
	Number	*%*
Classical Hippocratic only	5	3.9
Classical Hippocratic plus other	1	0.8
Modified Hippocratic only	42	32.8
Modified Hippocratic plus other	3	2.3
Declaration of Geneva only	30	23.4
Prayer of Maimonides only	9	7.0
Prayer of Maimonides plus other	2	1.6
Unknown oath	7	5.5
Other, only	16	12.5
No oath	13	10.2
TOTAL	128	100

Source: Friedlander, "Oaths Given by US and Canadian Medical Schools, 1977."
Note: Medical schools in the United States = 112; medical schools in Canada = 16; 94% US and 63% Canadians schools said they did administer an oath.

majority has rejected the Hippocratic form in favor of some other text or opted for no oath at all. Some of these alternative oaths come from modern professional organizations (the Declaration of Geneva), from individual physicians (Luis Lasagna), or from a school's religious tradition (the prayer named in honor of Maimonides). The Declaration of Geneva itself is historically connected to the Hippocratic Oath but includes many non-Hippocratic elements. No consistent or dominating pattern exists except the now total rejection of the original Hippocratic text.

Oath Taking, Weill Cornell Medical College, 2005

Confronted by the dissatisfaction with historical versions of the Hippocratic Oath, modern redrafts, and new oaths and pledges constructed by individuals or schools, some schools have taken it upon themselves to craft their own oath or pledge to be recited by their graduating classes. In some cases, each class has been invited to write its own oath each

Table 3.4   Use of Oaths in North American Medical Schools, 1993

	Medical Schools in the United States and Canada	
	Number	%
Used an oath	147	98
No oath	3	2
TOTAL	150	100
Classical Hippocratic Oath	1	0.7
Modern Hippocratic Oath	45	30.6
Modified Hippocratic Oath	22	15.0
Undesignated version of Hippocratic Oath	1	0.7
Declaration of Geneva	34	23.1
Prayer of Maimonides	4	2.7
Oath of Luis Lasagna	5	3.4
Osteopathic Oath	15	10.2
Other oath	20	13.6
TOTAL	147	100

Source: Orr, Pang, Pellegrino, and Siegler, "Use of the Hippocratic Oath."
Note: Medical schools in the United States = 135; medical schools in Canada = 15.

year, so it will emerge as an authentic product of the particular group of students. One effort by a school to create its own oath occurred at Weill Cornell Medical College in New York in 2005.

A committee appointed by the dean was formed under the leadership of Joseph Fins, a physician on the Cornell faculty and a recognized authority in medical ethics. The committee included twenty people—seventeen physicians, two medical students, and the director of pastoral care.[1] The resulting oath was probably as good as any generic pledge could be, but it raised serious issues. It is called the "Hippocratic Oath" and loosely follows some of the sentences of the original Oath, but it is significantly different in many respects.[2] Gone is most of the initial section that has an oath-of-initiation character to it. Gone also is the need to come to the financial aid of one's teachers or to consider their offspring as "equal to my brothers in male lineage." There is no restriction on sharing medical knowledge only with those who have taken the oath.

The code section is also dramatically different from the original Hippocratic document. There is no pledge to avoid abortion. No forswearing of giving deadly drugs. To the relief of students contemplating surgical specialization, there is no pledge to avoid surgery. Not only are the Greek gods and goddesses gone, but all religious reference vanishes. The Hippocratic virtues of purity and holiness are replaced with the virtues of "integrity" and "honor."[3] It is not clear why these are preferred to the AMA's "compassion" and "respect for human dignity." In their place are some very non-Hippocratic moral commitments: to "not withdraw from patients in their time of need," to "be an advocate for patients in need and strive for justice in the care of the sick," and to enter houses only for the good of the sick. It fudges on confidentiality in the same way the original oath does: swearing not to disclose those things that are "not fitting to be spoken," leaving the student to determine whether that would permit paternalistic breaches when the patient might not want information disclosed, or Tarasoff-like breaches to protect third parties even though disclosure might jeopardize the patient's welfare.

The writers note that the original oath seems harsh in threatening "retribution for any doctor who transgressed the oath and swore falsely."[4] It is replaced with a "more positive" ending in which the graduates "now turn to my calling, promising to preserve its finest traditions, with the reward of a long experience in the joy of healing."[5] This certainly means the graduate will escape the eternal damnation of failing to follow the original oath but still poses potential issues for some anti-Pelagians who believe that reward for good works is heretical.

This particular draft avoids some criticisms of the original oath but does so in part by finessing the difficult issues—euthanasia, abortion, the dilemma of the "Frankenstein myth," and the role of the clinician in rationing health care. It got at least one group of faculty and two students to take seriously the crafting of a set of pledges for the practice of medicine but did not address whether the rest of the 2005 graduating class or any future graduating classes are committed to its contents or even understand what they are promising. It seems doubtful that this oath can be taken by a graduate "solemnly," "freely," and "on my honor." One wonders what a graduate who disagrees with some of the provisions is to do.

The more fundamental problem remains. It seems unlikely that any one written document can adequately capture the ethical views of an entire group of students or even a majority of the group. Students come to medical school with religious and secular beliefs that differ. These beliefs will shape the student's understanding of the correct way to practice medicine. It is hard to believe that all students would concur with any single statement of the physician's duties—for or against abortion, for instance.

Even if by some miracle every student at Cornell was converted to the set of beliefs reflected in the local version of what they call their "Hippocratic Oath," these students will soon be practicing medicine with other interns and residents who have been coerced into participating in different graduation rituals that present them with different solemn oaths. And most critically, even if all of the students accepted this ethical statement, it is not clear that their patients would concur.

A Survey of Students at St. George's University School of Medicine in Grenada

To understand the nature of the commitments of a group of incoming medical students, my colleague, Cheryl Cox Macpherson, who teaches medical ethics with me at St. George's University School of Medicine, and I asked incoming medical students a series of questions during their first week at the school.[6] Along with the questions, we presented them with a standard list of the major religious, secular, and professional codes of ethics that a physician might use for guidance in the practice of medicine. We asked them:

> During the course of your medical practice you will inevitably face some difficult moral issues for which you may want some guidance and advice. One of the places you might turn for such advice might be various codes of medical ethics written by professional, religious, and/or governmental

groups. Below are 13 famous codes of medical ethics. Although you probably are not familiar with all of them, based on what you know today, which
one of these codes would be your first choice for such guidance?

Of the 364 students in the entering class, 289 answered our question.[7]
The results are presented in table 3.5.

The results were no doubt influenced by the fact that St. George's
is an international school drawing students for this class from forty-six
countries, but most came from the United States and an overwhelming
majority planned to practice medicine there. That no doubt led many
students to choose the AMA Code of Ethics, although barely half of

**Table 3.5 Student Choice of a Code for Moral Guidance (based on
current knowledge)**

Code Chosen by Student	Number	%
AMA Code of Ethics	149	51.6
BMA Code of Ethics	9	3.1
Ethical and Religious Directives for Catholic Health Facilities	5	1.7
Jewish Prayer of Maimonides and the Oath of Asaph	0	0.0
Hindu Caraka Samhita	2	0.7
Buddhist Seventeen Rules of Enjuin	4	1.4
American Hospital Association Patient's Bill of Rights	7	2.4
Islamic Code of Medical Ethics	3	1.0
Hippocratic Oath	56	19.4
World Medical Association's Declaration of Geneva	19	6.6
Russian Oath for Physicians (1992)	0	0.0
UNESCO's Universal Declaration on Bioethics and Human Rights	17	5.9
St. George's University Academic Oath	5	1.7
Other	13	4.5
TOTAL	289	100

Source: Veatch and Macpherson, "Medical School Oath-Taking," 339.

Note: Other = Don't know/blank, 4; Sikh, 1; Jesus first, 1; all seem reasonable, 1; British
Columbia Medical Association, 1; Canadian Medical Association, 1; personal reflection, 2;
the patient and her religious community, 1; the Bible, 1.

them made that choice. It is striking that only 5 out of 289 selected the school's academic oath—the oath they all would be asked to swear less than four years later when they would graduate.

The repeat of the question following the third term, when the ethics instruction at the school had been completed, produced a much smaller response from a group of students who were now deeply engrossed in their studies and under no pressure to complete the repeat survey. Of seventy-eight who completed the question, thirty-seven changed their choice of a code they would choose for guidance, but no clear pattern emerged. Seventeen changed from the Hippocratic Oath; six from the World Medical Association Declaration of Geneva; and four from the AMA to some other code. The St. George's Academic Oath gained six adherents but lost one of its original supporters. If the school were to impose any one codification on its entire graduating class, the most plausible choice would appear to be the AMA Code, but even that would conflict with the student's choice nearly half the time. Clearly, almost all the students still preferred some option other than the school's own oath.

This posed a significant problem for the faculty of a health professional school responsible for teaching ethics. We now knew that the students who were going to be handed a piece of paper and asked to recite the St. George's Academic Oath would, at the point about halfway through their education and after they had received exposure to the St. George's Academic Oath, still almost all choose something else and, although the AMA Code was preferred by about half the students, there was no clear consensus on any one document. Some religious students still preferred their own religious documents; secular students (as well as many who acknowledged association with some religious tradition) still preferred some national or international codification coming either from a professional or a lay group.

Students were going to be placed in the awkward position of being expected to participate in a graduation ritual in which they would solemnly swear to a document when they, in fact, had other preferences. The St. George's Academic Oath represents a modern, relatively innocuous code rather similar to the Weill Cornell Oath in many ways. Still, it was not without controversy. It includes swearing by "Almighty God," which could offend some people. It deletes most of the archaic Hippocratic conditions (such as duties to professors and the prohibition on surgery) but retains a provision that students will be "ever faithful to St. George's University" and a closing prayer that God help the student keep the oath and that, if the graduate does, she will gain "respect by all men in all times." It contains an odd provision that seems to be the replacement for the Hippocratic prohibition on giving deadly drugs. It has the student pledge not "maliciously to cause the death of anyone," of course, leaving open the ethically challenging question of whether a physician may benevolently cause anyone's death. This has all the marks of code by committee in which some wanted to forswear all killing by physicians including mercy killings while others wanted to remain open to merciful killings but were willing to agree to prohibit malicious ones.

Surely, some Catholic, Jewish, and Muslim students would have wanted a stronger antikilling pledge, and just as surely, some student who was sympathetic with Jack Kevorkian would have wanted to acknowledge the legitimacy of some mercy killings. Muslim students, of which there were many, would presumably find an oath taken in the name of Allah with support from the Qur'an more meaningful. Atheists would presumably prefer to get rid of the references to the deity.

Students have asked me what they should do if they disagree with parts of the St. George's Oath. Their options are limited. They could remain silent hoping others would not notice. They could cross their fingers behind their backs, a time-honored device for making promises that do not count. They could refuse to attend the graduation ceremony. They could ask for a reconsideration of whether the recitation should be included in the ceremony.

Some defenders of commencement oath taking have responded to this concern by claiming that the ritual of reciting a so-called solemn oath is merely a time-honored symbol of entry into a new stage of life or into a new professional relationship and that one should not be concerned about the literal content of the oath. That is a troublesome response on two counts.

First, it seems odd that the position of either faculty or students should be that solemn promises explicitly in the realm of ethics could be ignored and do not really count as promises. Having the graduating medical student commit, in his first act as a professional, to a promise he does not take seriously and does not intend to keep is odd indeed.

Second, one could question at an even more basic level whether it is good for students to enter into a ritual symbolizing that they are leaving one set of cultural and institutional commitments and entering another. Some medical students will still be members of religious groups and expected to base their ethics on the positions of those groups. Others will remain secular adherents to basic philosophical movements—liberal political philosophy, libertarianism, feminism, socialism, and the like. It is problematic to suggest that entry into a profession must be accompanied by a correlative lessening of the ties to the traditional groups that provide the foundation of the newly minted physician's set of moral commitments.

Claiming one is not lessening these traditional commitments but merely adding a new one doesn't seem defensible either. On matters of morality, professional sources are in direct competition with religious and philosophical sources. One cannot claim simultaneously that the norms by which one practices one's craft come from two diverse and sometimes contradictory foundations. If one's religious or philosophical commitments include commitment to moral norms requiring one set of behaviors, one cannot simultaneously profess loyalty to another set of commitments coming from another source such as a school or professional group. After examining the limits of professionally generated codes of ethics in the following chapter, we will examine in detail how the ethical systems grounded in religion and philosophy exert their claim on the adherents to those movements.

The Implications of Medical School Oath Taking

The patterns of medical school oath taking pose serious issues. It is clear that, at least since the beginning of the twentieth century, only a very small minority of North American medical students have taken the Hippocratic Oath upon graduation. Given the almost complete absence of interest in the Oath prior to that time, it seems obvious this is also true of North American students prior to that time. Thus, any assumption that the ethical duties of physicians are based in their having taken the Hippocratic Oath on graduation from medical schools is mistaken. More troubling, there is no alternative professional oath that can muster a clear consensus. Any other single pledge by physicians is not only absent in the history of the profession of medicine; it is not plausible as a goal for the future. If St. George's University is any indication, none of the options musters more than a bare majority. Surely there is no oath or pledge of professional ethics that a majority has taken. This means that, when patients encounter physicians in practice, they cannot assume that the physician is committed to any one professional oath. Moreover, since the students have graduated from many different schools, when physicians practice as a group (in a group practice, an HMO, or a hospital) they would be pledged to different codes. If they take their medical school commitment seriously, they have different moral commitments.

Most critically, even if we could discern what code commanded the loyalty of the physician, there is no reason to assume that the patient would share that vision of the moral standards for professional conduct. Even on the issues that will affect the way the patient is treated, the patient has no voice. For example, the ethical standards for when a physician can conduct medical research on a patient without informing the patient would be outside the influence of the patient. Since most of the medical school oaths or pledges or codes were crafted by some professional or student group, the patients were not a party to the creation of the content of these commitments. There is no reason to believe that they represent the patients' moral understanding of the ethics that should govern the relation between provider and patient. Most dramatically, there is no reason they should govern when patients should be obligated to concur in the decisions of physicians or surrender their rights such as the right to refuse to agree to proposed treatments. In short, to the extent that medical school pledges are taken seriously—and perhaps they should not be—a patient cannot assume that the physician's commitment was to the Hippocratic Oath. Moreover, the patient has no basis for assuming any other professionally generated moral pledge was taken. Even if some enterprising patient researched the physician's school and determined that some particular oath was taken, the patient is unlikely to share the moral commitments of that document and has reason to suspect that the physician doesn't either.

We need to think more clearly about whether it is a good thing for those being socialized into a profession to be led to believe they are set apart and no longer part of their preprofessional groups. The time for professional oath taking is over. Such oaths should be abandoned in favor of commitments of the professional grounded outside the profession.

4

THE LIMITS OF
PROFESSIONALLY
GENERATED ETHICS

T HE HIPPOCRATIC ETHICAL TRADITION and the other professionally generated codes of medical ethics that have arisen as
alternatives leave the world of medical ethics with a very unsat-
isfying set of options. One could attempt to revise the Oath. As we have
seen, many medical schools have attempted that but have failed to
achieve a satisfying revision. Alternatively, a new and different professionally generated code could be developed. In this chapter we see the
problems with that approach and look at three examples of the kinds
of difficulties codes written by professional groups have caused. In the
following chapters we turn to the alternatives of religious and secular
philosophical sources of an ethic for the health professions.

Alternative Professionally Generated Ethics

The alternative professionally generated ethics, such as the AMA code
of 1847, are not as offensive in claiming that their knowledge of the
ethical norms for physicians is an esoteric secret. These ethics are more

public in their ethics generation than were the members of the Philadelphia Kappa Lambda fraternity. Any member of the public can buy a copy of the current *Code of Ethics of the American Medical Association* (although laypeople have to pay a surcharge). The AMA still presumes, however, that only the physician group can play a role in articulating the code of ethics that governs the group's members' relations with patients.

Modern and postmodern physicians are in an awkward position. Many see themselves as standing in some religious tradition. They are faithful communicants in Christian churches, members of synagogues, or, increasingly, Muslims or people who stand in family traditions with Asian heritage that they perceive as still shaping their moral worldviews. Once one grants that professional groups are claiming a role in generating or articulating codes of ethics, those professional groups must be perceived competitors with the religious communities that also claim they are the mediators of moral norms, whether through revelation, scripture, or authoritative interpretation of the natural law. One cannot subscribe to the professional role in generating codes of moral norms for physicians in their interactions with patients and simultaneously endorse the metaethics of a major religious community.

Physicians who see themselves as part of the tradition of secular liberal political philosophy or some other secular philosophical tradition face a similar problem. They cannot simultaneously accept the metaethical theories of one of the major secular philosophical traditions, complete with their claims that ethics is known through reason, empirical understanding, or social contract, and continue to give professional groups a privileged place in generating or articulating the norms for physicians. One cannot simultaneously be committed to the metaethic of the profession and the metaethic of a secular philosophical tradition.

The puzzle is why a professional group would claim authority to articulate a set of moral norms or a moral code for its members. The problem is particularly acute when the norms being articulated govern relations between members of the professional group and patients who are not normally members of that group. Because patients are not part of the profession, their fate will be placed in the hands of a group of people who do not share the moral perspective of the patient, and who claim that their group has the capacity and authority to determine the norms that govern the way patients will be treated.

An Internal Morality for Medicine

One defense of having a medical faculty or professional group generate or articulate a code of ethics for its members (including norms that are intended to govern conduct between members and patients who are not members) is that the very concept of medicine contains within it a set of moral imperatives that must apply to all members of the profession of medicine. The claim is that a morality internal to the professional practice can be discerned by careful reflection on the very concepts of medicine and health.[1] The claim is that the very nature of medicine is to heal and that the duty of the physician or other health professional can be derived from understanding what it means to heal. There are three major problems with this claim, however.

Laypeople Should Be Able to Contribute to a Discussion of What It Means to Heal

First, even if one could establish the moral norms for the healer by the power of reflection on what it means to heal, it is not clear why only members of the healing profession should be able to carry out such reflection. The most astute proponent of the internal morality thesis, my friend and colleague Edmund D. Pellegrino, readily acknowledges this.[2]

Proponents of this teleological approach to discerning the norms for the healer claim that there are natural ends appropriate to such roles, ends the knowledge of which is available by the brute analysis of the roles themselves. But there is no reason why only those professionally committed to one of these roles should be able to understand what it means to heal and what the natural end of healing is. Patients, familial surrogates, public policymakers, and academics in theology and philosophy all ought to be able to carry out such analysis.

One might concede that those who think a great deal about the healing role might have more insight into that role than those who encounter the issue only in passing and perhaps only in moments of crisis. Nevertheless, not all healing professionals do think often and hard about the ends they are pursuing, and certainly many who are not healing professionals—academics, for instance—may do so.

More critically, it could be that those approaching this teleological task from different perspectives may come up with somewhat differing insights. Thus, clinicians who spend all their days over a long career caring for patients may have a somewhat different understanding of the role than an academic physician, a theologian who teaches pastoral care, or a scholar expert in the history of medicine. A physician in the military may think differently about the ends of healing than does a physician who is a member of Doctors without Borders, and each may think differently about the healing role than did Jack Kevorkian. Chronically ill patients may have still another understanding of the nature of healing. At the very least, the internal morality thesis provides no support for the claim that teachers of medicine or careerists in organized medicine have the unique authority to discern the role of the healer and the norms that the role implies.

Using the Medical Profession for Nonmedical Purposes

Second, it may be that society wishes to use its professionally competent practitioners from time to time for good purposes that are nevertheless nonmedical. Members of the society might need medical interventions to provide benefits that are not in the medical domain and do not involve healing but are important social objectives nevertheless. Some of these nonmedical social purposes may be morally controversial. They may involve controlling fertility and abortion, ending life humanely, changing physical appearance, or enhancing athletic ability. The defenders of the internal morality of medicine position claim that these activities are not part of healing and are thus not part of the essence of being a physician.

To be sure, some of these purposes may be morally suspect. Many people oppose abortion, euthanasia, or the use of performance-enhancing drugs to gain an advantage in a sports competition. The issue, however, is whether it is the medical profession's place to decide whether these activities are worthwhile or immoral and whether physicians should be used for these purposes.

Some nonhealing activities that require highly complex medical skills may be morally worthwhile—indeed, good ends to pursue. Others surely are not. Consider, for example, the difficult problem of military pilots who are sometimes required to fly very long missions in small planes that can contain only one pilot.[3] Assuming there are some military missions that are morally justifiable, it can be critical that such pilots maintain heightened states of alertness for perhaps as long as twenty-four hours. This is not reasonable for normal humans unaided by medical support, but this could be made more feasible by performance-enhancing medical interventions. If these interventions are justified, they are justified on military, political, or social grounds, yet surely highly skilled medical professionals should be among the ones involved in planning such interventions. It seems wrong to claim that, since the goal is not medical and certainly does not involve "healing," the task is outside the domain of physician responsibility. Whether the task is a healing task is not critical. Whether the objective is defensible and requires the skill of a medical professional is what matters.

Society has a right to decide whether these activities are acceptable or should be banned, but it is not clear why the medical profession should be in the position to make those judgments or why the determination of whether the end is medical should establish the legitimacy of physician participation. We can imagine other important social purposes that would require a medical enhancement of someone's skills in order to achieve maximal success. A firefighter who could perform at superhuman levels if he or she received a performance-enhancing medical intervention may save lives or accomplish important social goals. The simple device of an oxygen mask might be an example. If medical expertise is needed to determine the proper settings on the oxygen mask, surely it makes no difference whether the task is classified as a healing one. Even if it is not, the objective seems important, and physician participation is certainly warranted, if needed. It is not clear why it should be up to the medical profession to determine whether these medical interventions for nonmedical purposes should be justified.

Insofar as the license to practice medicine provides a socially conveyed authority, it seems reasonable that the society, not the profession, should be the authority to determine whether it is acceptable for licensed health professionals to provide such services. The same argument arises in other social projects requiring professional medical skill: capital punishment (discussed later), cosmetic surgery, performance enhancement in sports, and monitoring the safety of boxers or football players, for example. It is not a matter of whether the intervention is for the end of healing. If the intervention is worthwhile and is complex enough that it requires the skill of a licensed professional to provide it safely, then whether it counts as healing or is in any other way implied in the concepts of medicine or health should not matter.

Determining What It Means to Heal

Third, even within the realm of healing, normative judgments must be made. Merely to determine exactly what it means to heal requires an appeal beyond the profession of medicine. The concept of healing does not provide inherent guidance on how to promote the well-being of the human in the medical sphere. The members of a profession attempting to add content to their understanding of what it means to heal must turn outside of the profession for answers to critical questions about the purpose of the profession.

For example, if healing is (one of) the goals of the profession of medicine, we need to ask precisely what it means to heal. Answers to that question will be forthcoming from various religious and secular philosophical worldviews. Consider the increasingly important question of whether medicine has, as part of its central mission, the extension of the normal life span beyond the historical three score and ten.

Since the 1970s we have understood that medicine can have two separate potential functions related to how long people live.[4] We have long recognized that some people have medical problems that will end their lives prematurely if an intervention does not correct what is wrong. A person may have a lethal infection, a genetic disease, or an anatomical structure that means that the person will not live out what we take to be a normal life span—traditionally thought of as about seventy or eighty years. Everyone easily recognizes that professionals in medicine have the ability to correct these problems that can cut a life short.

However, what about interventions that take the person who is on track to live the normal life span and extend that person's life some additional years? Various theories attempt to account for this idea of each species having a normal life span to which members of the species will live unless they are cut down early by disease.[5] Perhaps a genetic or other biological clock runs down after a normal number of years. The issue is whether attempts to modify the normal aging process should count as healing or as abnormally enhancing a natural limit in human functioning. All the reflection in the world by members of the medical profession on the concept of healing would not seem to be able to answer a question such as this. Mere deep thinking about what it means to heal leaves us uncertain about whether changing a natural limit in the human organism would count as healing or enhancement.[6] Some would claim that it really does not matter whether it is called healing or not; the real issue is whether such a change in the nature of the species—such a "resetting of the biological clock"—is morally legitimate or is human hubris. Thinking about healing will not answer this kind of question. This is the kind of question that a medical professional group would seem to have no inherent right to answer and no grounds for answering. It is the kind of question on which religious worldviews or secular equivalents might more appropriately contribute.

Thus, even if for some reason we decide that medical professionals should be limited in their professional activity to something called healing, there is no internal vantage point within the professional group or the medical school oath writers for deciding whether many potential interventions should count as healing. There is no reason to assume that merely because one is a member of a profession of healers one should know what activities are within that profession's domain. Jewish physicians, radical feminist physicians, Nazi physicians, Marxist physicians, and physicians whose worldviews are shaped by liberal political philosophy will reasonably have different understandings both of what it means to heal and of whether the work of physicians and other health professionals should extend beyond healing to important social functions that are not medical. It is impossible to know the ends of medicine without looking outside medicine to some worldview. The alternatives are normally articulated by religions or secular analogues. The medical profession and its educators cannot function as a source for a consistent worldview about what ends are worth pursuing in life that would seem appropriate to all physicians. Even if it could, patients and other medical laypeople are, by definition, not part of that group and should not be expected to accept the professional group's conclusions.

Pellegrino and others who are more sophisticated in their appeal to an internal morality for medicine as a basis for determining the duties of the medical professional recognize that reflection on the concepts of medicine and healing need not be restricted to members of the professional group. Medical laypeople, including philosophers, theologians, and ordinary citizens, also may think about these concepts and attempt to deduce the ends that health professionals ought to pursue.

Even granting that these activities are fair game for those who are not members of the profession leaves serious problems, however. If the bare concepts of medicine and healing cannot provide the critical content without appeal outside of medicine to basic systems of religious and philosophical belief, then we must acknowledge that the real grounds for professional duty are necessarily external to the profession. Neither professionals nor laypeople can know the proper ends of a profession without looking beyond the profession.

Pellegrino is richly schooled in Roman Catholic moral theology and classical philosophy. He understands well the teleological natural law system that places limits on the conduct of both health professionals and laypeople. He derives his teleological worldview from these religious and philosophical sources, which he believes are accessible to some extent based on reason and therefore accessible to all persons, whether they are Catholic or not and whether they are physicians or not. To understand the ends of the medical professional, he would logically ask what the ends of human existence are—a question for him appropriately answered by natural law theory guided by the theological and philosophical wisdom of the "doctors of the church" (that is, its theologians) and other standard sources of wisdom (such as the philosophers of ancient Greece). Logically, the defender of such a worldview should be committed to understanding the ends of medicine (and therefore the ends of the medical professional) by looking to sources external to medicine—that is, the most fundamental understanding of human ends articulated by the belief system's traditional sources of authority. Likewise, members of other religious and philosophical traditions would appropriately be committed to turning to their sources of authority external to medicine to understand the ends of medicine and the moral limits on the practice of the various professions as seen by their worldview. If, and only if, there is hope for some convergence of the various worldviews about the nature of the various professions, then is there hope for convergence about the moral norms for practicing those professions that should extend beyond sectarian commitment.

Some examples may help illustrate the problem. Let us consider three: nutrition and hydration, capital punishment, and surrogate motherhood.

Nutrition and Hydration

A medical ethical dilemma arises when critically or terminally ill patients are being provided nutrition and hydration by medical means. Some patients are chronically ill and stable, perhaps in a coma or a vegetative state. The famous case of Terri Schiavo is only one dramatic example.[7] In the United States many cases involving such patients have led to disputes over whether it is morally acceptable to withdraw nutrition and hydration when it is determined that the patient, who may or may not be conscious, will not suffer and is getting no benefit from these treatments.

Some people believe that nutrition and hydration are basic care that must always be provided.[8] Others defend the provision of these treatments because they are seen as socially important symbols of society's commitment to those who are at risk for hunger or thirst.[9] On the other hand, many people believe that the only reason to provide nutrition and hydration is to serve some useful purpose and that, therefore, it is appropriately forgone in cases when no benefit is anticipated. Patients for whom such decisions are to be made may be terminally ill or merely chronically ill but not terminal. Patients may be permanently unconscious or may retain some potential for consciousness. Deciding exactly when, if ever, nutrition and hydration may be withheld is a complex, controversial task about which people and groups disagree.

The issue is whether the professional group is the appropriate locus for resolving such moral conflicts. The Hippocratic Oath is not of much help. It speaks more generally, and this specific issue had not yet arisen when the Oath was written. However, professional groups can formulate a position on these questions, perhaps claiming that their position is their interpretation of the Oath or of some other moral foundation.

For example, the American Medical Association has specifically addressed the issue of providing nutrition and hydration for critically and terminally ill patients. For a time in the late 1980s and early 1990s, when these issues were particularly controversial, the AMA endorsed a policy of discontinuing all means of life-prolonging medical treatment including artificially or technologically supplied nutrition or hydration when death was imminent or the patient was "beyond doubt permanently unconscious."[10] It also claimed, however, that "unless it is clearly established that the patient is terminally ill or permanently unconscious, a physician should not be deterred from appropriately aggressive treatment of a patient,"[11] a statement uniformly understood to require nutrition and hydration for patients who were not terminally ill or permanently unconscious. The AMA's policy seems on its face to even require the physician to provide nutrition and hydration for someone who is quite probably permanently unconscious but could possibly recover to what is now being called "a minimally conscious state." Such a person would not ever recover full consciousness or even the capacity to voluntarily control bodily movement. The person would still be permanently immobile and bedridden, unable to communicate, but possibly able to perceive small amounts of sensation (including pain).

It seems plausible that some such people and their surrogates may still choose to withdraw nutrition and hydration on the grounds that they do not offer proportional benefit. If the individual may actually be minimally conscious, that adds the additional possibility that the person may be suffering. Nevertheless, because the patient is not "beyond doubt permanently unconscious," the AMA took the position that its members should not be deterred from providing aggressive treatment. This position of the AMA was in conflict both with conservative groups who insisted on providing medical means of nutrition and hydration in all cases (including terminal illness and permanent unconsciousness) and with more liberal groups that supported withholding nutrition and hydration in certain cases in which the patient may be critically ill but neither terminal nor permanently unconscious (such as the minimally conscious state with the possibility of suffering).

At issue, then, is how a physician should act when his professional group holds that nutrition and hydration should be provided while he or she is a member of a religious or secular group that condones withholding it. A physician may be a Roman Catholic, for example. The Catholic Church generally defends a duty to provide nutrition and hydration but accepts withholding it in special cases in which the treatment would be burdensome or provide no benefit.[12] Thus, a Catholic physician may be advised by the Church that it is acceptable to withhold treatment, while his professional group may be telling him that it should be provided.

An even more complex problem can arise if the physician is a member of a religious group that insists it is morally necessary to provide nutrition and hydration even if the patient is terminally ill or permanently unconscious. For example, some Orthodox Jews would insist on providing such support regardless of terminal illness or permanent unconsciousness. In that case, the physician's religious guidance would require treatment while her medical professional group would not require it. The secular society and its legal structures might have still another position. Is there any reason to assume that the professional group should be definitive in these cases?

In all of these situations the patient's religious or secular community may also have positions on these matters so that physicians' guidance from the professional association may be in conflict not only with their own religious and secular worldviews but also with the worldview of the patient. It seems odd indeed that the professional group's guidance of the moment should be seen as definitive.

This example is made even more complex with the modification in 1994 of the AMA position. At that time, the AMA removed the language suggesting a duty to provide aggressive life support in all cases in which the patient is neither terminal nor permanently unconscious. Now, a valid refusal by the patient or surrogate is given more respect. Now it is "not unethical" to withhold such treatments based on the patient's wishes.[13] Is it really sensible to hold that, during the period (but only during this period) when the AMA required aggressive life support for the patient who was neither terminally ill nor unconscious, it was morally right for the physician to provide it even when the patient, supported by her religious or secular worldview and by the laws of the state, insisted it should not be provided?

Capital Punishment

A second example of how professional groups compete with religious and secular systems of belief and values arises in the area of capital punishment. The AMA has taken a strong stand against participation of physicians in capital punishment.[14] The issue arises more directly as a society shifts, for reasons of humaneness, to medical means of execution and away from more barbaric forms such as electrocution. Even though electrocution was once itself advocated for its relative gentleness (compared with the guillotine or hanging), considerable support emerged in the twentieth century for medical means that would simply "put the prisoner to sleep"—permanently. The World Medical Association has taken a very similar stance in opposition to physician participation in these medical means of execution, as does the British Medical Association.[15]

With medicalization of capital punishment comes many points of contact for the medical professional. It is not likely that the physician would be in the position of actual executioner, but a trained medical professional could be given many roles related to an execution: advising on the drugs to be used, calculating the proper drug dosages, preparing the prisoner, and perhaps placing an IV line that would later be used for administration of the lethal agent. The physician could monitor for failure of the drugs to do their intended job, could monitor for the moment of death, pronounce death, and so forth. The issue is whether it is ethical for the physician to play any of these roles.

The AMA has taken a strong stand that any such behaviors are contrary to the nature of being a physician:

> A physician, as a member of a profession dedicated to preserving life when there is hope of doing so, should not be a participant in a legally authorized execution. . . . Physician participation in execution includes, but is not limited to, the following actions: prescribing or administering tranquilizers and other psychotropic agents and medications that are part of the execution procedure; monitoring vital signs on site or remotely (including monitoring electrocardiograms); attending or observing an execution as a physician; and rendering of technical advice regarding execution.[16]

The AMA even goes to the extreme of defining some behaviors related to the criminal scheduled for execution that are morally acceptable for the physician, such as testifying about the criminal's medical history and diagnosis or mental state, or about relevant medical evidence, certifying death. The physician, according to the AMA, may also witness an execution "in a totally nonprofessional capacity" at the voluntary request of the prisoner, provided that such witness is in a "nonprofessional capacity."[17]

He or she may also relieve "acute suffering of a condemned person while awaiting execution, including providing tranquilizers at the specific voluntary request of the condemned person to help relieve pain or anxiety in anticipation of the execution."[18]

Thus, the AMA sees fit to pronounce on momentous moral aspects of a major controversial public matter, even opining on what is ethical in the physician's nonprofessional capacity. The puzzle is why in the world a medical professional organization would feel it has the authority to take positions on such matters. To be sure, the issue, at least until one turns to nonprofessional behaviors, involves the role of the medical professional and organized medical professional organizations have traditionally claimed authority in deciding what constitutes ethically appropriate behavior for people in the professional role. Why, however, would a collectivity of people in a role have this kind of authority; why would they claim hegemony over the moral norms for people in that role?

The American Board of Anesthesiology (ABA) seems to go even further. It explicitly endorses the AMA position that physicians cannot participate in capital punishment, but it then commits to the possibility of revoking board diplomate status of any anesthesiologist who chooses to participate. It holds: "If diplomates of the ABA participate in an execution by lethal injection, they may be subject to disciplinary action, including revocation of their ABA diplomate status."[19]

The ABA goes on to make a remarkable distinction. A commentary on the ABA policy regarding capital punishment written by Mark A. Rockoff, the secretary of the ABA, and dated April 2, 2010, makes clear that the ABA is not taking a position on the practice of capital punishment, just on the participation of anesthesiologists in the practice as members of their profession. "The ABA has not taken this action because of any position regarding the appropriateness of the death penalty. Anesthesiologists, like all physicians and all citizens, have different personal opinions about capital punishment. Nonetheless, the ABA, like the AMA, believes strongly that physicians should not be involved in capital punishment."[20]

Thus, the ABA acknowledges that people will have a range of views on capital punishment and that the professional association cannot claim expertise on the legitimacy of the practice. Nevertheless, the ABA believes it can claim authority to conclude that those trained in anesthesiology and given diplomate status by their group cannot participate ethically. In effect, they claim custody of anyone who has been certified as having professional standing in anesthesiology even though they admit they cannot claim expertise on the practice of capital punishment itself.

The problem here is that the practice of capital punishment is, as the ABA admits, a matter of public policy and, thus, for society to decide. Individuals within society must formulate a judgment on this ethical question. Some citizens and some courts have determined that execution by medical means is the most ethical way to carry out a death sentence and that the participation of people with appropriate medical knowledge is critical. The questions, then, are whether there is anything about being an anesthesiologist that should rightly exclude those who have decided it is appropriate to participate in executions, and whether the ABA is justified in prohibiting anesthesiologists who have made such a decision from following their consciences and the teachings of their religious or cultural affiliates.

I find no moral justification for capital punishment in a world in which human life is precious. Errors are increasingly documented in establishing the guilt of those charged with capital offenses as well as in determining whether the convicted are mentally responsible for their behavior. I would therefore lobby for the policy that exists in some states to prohibit all executions as cruel and too irreversible to be considered fair in a society known to make serious errors. But the issue here is whether a state that has chosen, after deliberation, to continue executing its criminals and has determined that execution by medical means is the most humane method should have the authority to require the presence of a medically competent professional. If so, does a private professional organization whose task is to certify professional competency also have the right to specify the moral standards under which technically competent physicians may practice their craft?

The professional group is sometimes believed to create the role of the medical professional. That is surely a mistake, however. Rather, that role comes from a far more fundamental foundation. As a matter of public policy, the responsibility rests with the society that sees fit to establish lay and professional roles and to license professional practitioners deemed capable of fulfilling that role. Since the role will have moral as well as technical limits, it is the society—not the professional association—that legitimately has the authority to define the ethical standards under which the role is carried out. Presumably, a state that has seen fit to continue the barbaric practice of capital punishment and then insists that technically competent professionals be present to ensure that the practice is carried out competently would define the professional role so that at least some who fulfill that role would be permitted to participate in the deadly deed.

Because only a very small number of physicians are needed for this capital punishment role and thus far competent members of the profession have been willing to step forward to perform this tragic task, it makes sense that no physician should be required to participate against his or her will. There is, however, no basis for the professional association to prohibit its diplomates from participating. There is nothing about being a member of the professional group that gives the group sole custody of the moral norms governing state-licensed physicians who are members of the profession. That is the role of the state. As long as some states see fit to continue capital punishment, willing members of the profession should be permitted to participate and, indeed, requiring some willing member to be present seems wise if the practice is to continue.

Physicians are simultaneously members of religious, philosophical, or cultural groups that also claim such authority. A physician who is also a Catholic or a Southern Baptist or a democratic socialist might turn to his religious or philosophical group to get guidance on whether physicians should participate in executions, or he might turn to organized medicine. Most people would understand if a physician were to say she cannot participate in an execution because she is a Catholic and the Church's moral theology opposes execution. In fact, the Catholic Church has repeatedly affirmed its opposition to the death penalty.[21] Often their opposition is expressed theologically as part of what has been called the "seamless garment argument," the view that the Church is pro-life and that defense of life must be seamless from the prenatal period to the end of life.[22]

One might also understand if a physician was to say that he is a Southern Baptist and, as such, he follows his church's interpretation of biblical teaching, which supports justice through the use of the death penalty. His church has said that "the messengers to the Southern Baptist Convention, meeting in Orlando, Florida, June 13 [and] 14, 2000, support the fair and equitable use of capital punishment by civil magistrates as a legitimate form of punishment for those guilty of murder or treasonous acts that result in death."[23]

Of course, no member of the Catholic or Southern Baptist churches will automatically adopt the church's position on social ethical matters including capital punishment, but one can understand that, by the time a member of one of these traditions accepts the theological premises of the group (including its claims to be authoritative on matters of morality), it would not be surprising if the individual who has chosen to become a loyal member of the particular church would share many of its positions and the reasons for those positions.

Likewise, physicians who are mainstream Protestants are likely to share their churches' opposition to the death penalty; Missouri Synod Lutherans and at least some Jews and Muslims are likely to defend it.[24] Similarly, those who stand in various philosophical traditions that have developed positions will no doubt be influenced by their belief systems. ACLU members may give traditional civil liberties arguments against it.[25] The Republican Party platform has supported it.[26]

In contrast with these religious and secular groups that have well-developed metaethical systems that lead them to adopt certain positions on moral issues including capital punishment, it is not clear why a complex collective organization of those who practice medicine should be led to one position or another on participation in capital punishment. The historical values of medicine have supported physicians who take actions to relieve suffering. Medical execution is surely a lessening of suffering compared with traditional, more violent executions. On the other hand, the historical values of medicine have supported physicians who oppose death. The Hippocratic Oath opposed giving a deadly drug even if asked for it. The exact meaning has never been clear—whether it implies opposition to mercy killing or conspiring to commit homicide at the request of someone's enemy. Moreover, the Oath does not condemn placing IV lines, calculating doses, supervising injections, or pronouncing death. It certainly does not advise on what a physician should do if she sees someone suffering because an attempt at execution has been botched.

One could imagine church members or members of secular advocacy organizations having views on these possible physician activities. One can for the same reasons imagine members who are also physicians having relevant views. But on what grounds could the mere fact that one is a physician—independent of one's moral and religious views—lead one to favor or oppose capital punishment?

Presumably, some who have chosen the career of physician will have developed moral views coming down in favor of capital punishment; some will have developed moral views opposed. There is no reason why all physicians regardless of their moral, religious, and philosophical views would come down exactly the same way. Then why would we expect all members of the AMA or the ABA to have consistent and rational views unless, for some reason, all its members came from moral traditions with consistent views on the subject? The mere fact that the sociological process of becoming a physician led to the outcome that more physicians favored one view than favored another surely is not reason enough to expect all physicians to reach the same conclusion or for the minority to yield to the majority position. Nothing about being a physician should give medical professional groups epistemological authority over moral matters. Nothing in the expertise of being a physician gives one expertise in making moral judgments.

Not surprisingly, when capital punishment debates occur in state legislatures, physicians end up on both sides of the argument. In California, for example, in response to a controversy over physician involvement in executions, Assemblyman Alan Nakanishi, an eye surgeon, introduced a bill sponsored by the California Medical Association prohibiting physician participation in executions. Meanwhile, another state senator who happened to be a general anesthesiologist, Sam Aanestad, introduced legislation to protect physicians who participate in executions from punishment or professional discipline.

It is hard to see why the California Medical Association should weigh in on the side of a physician attempting to exclude physicians rather than on the side of the physician attempting to protect physicians who thought participation was the right choice. One might easily give reasons on one side or the other that are grounded in religious or philosophical positions for or against capital punishment. It is harder to see why physicians, as a group, ought to come to one or another of the moral positions unless, by chance, they are made up of a majority happening to stand in one or the other tradition.

Surrogate Motherhood

A third example of organized medicine taking a controversial position on a matter of morality is found in surrogate motherhood. As described by the AMA, surrogacy involves artificial insemination of a woman who agrees to carry a fetus to term and surrender parental rights, usually to the father of the child who supplied the sperm for the insemination. In cases of gestational surrogacy, the woman is impregnated with an in vitro fertilized egg, typically from the spouse of the man who is the source of the sperm. In this case, the couple supplying the egg and sperm cells typically intends to assume parental rights and responsibilities.

Such practices raise complex moral, legal, and practical controversies, and it is not surprising that different religious and secular groups take differing positions. The Catholic Church, as expected, opposes the practice, counting it an unnatural manipulation of the birth process. It is also opposed by some feminist groups on grounds that it is an abuse of the gestating woman who should not be "used" as a mere incubator and should not be forced to agree to surrender parenting rights since she has no way of knowing the emotional bonding that can take place during pregnancy. Likewise, some groups object to the interconnecting of the birth process with financial and legal obligations.

On the other hand, pronatalist groups might support surrogacy as the most reliable way of permitting infertile persons or couples to have children that are at least partly genetically their own. Libertarians support the right of mentally competent adults to make binding agreements that advance mutual interests and object to legal interference with the right to contract. They claim that prohibiting a woman from making such an arrangement is demeaning to her since it implies she is not capable of rational planning to pursue her own interests or her own sense of charity.

People influenced by differing religious, philosophical, and cultural groups could develop complex and conflicting positions on surrogacy. On the other hand, a group of medical professionals drawn from this range of differing religious, philosophical, and cultural groups are unlikely to form a consensus opinion on the morality of surrogacy. Nevertheless, that is what the AMA has done. It holds that surrogacy contracts are permissible (a position that should offend Catholic physicians who accept traditional natural law views on conception) but that it should be legal for the surrogate mother to "void the contract within a reasonable period of time after the birth of the child"[27] (a position that might please some militant feminists but should offend libertarians who support the moral right to form contracts and the moral obligation to keep them once they are formed).

No grounds exist on which an organized collective of medical professionals made up of men and women coming from every imaginable religious, philosophical, and cultural perspective could form a consensus on this set of questions. No metaethical theory exists upon which an eclectic group of professionals bound together only by their common professional discipline should be able to reach such a consensus. One needs a claim to authority on the foundation or grounding of morality in order to claim expertise in matters of ethics. That is precisely what religions and philosophical schools of thought claim. There is no plausible grounds upon which the mere gathering together of those with professional-level expertise in medicine (or law or accounting or any other profession) can claim expertise on the grounding of morality. Those who have been socialized into a profession learn to master a craft with all the technical knowledge and skill that is required. Knowing all there is to know about one's profession, however, does not give one expertise on questions of morality—whether it is acceptable to withhold nutrition from certain dying humans, whether it is appropriate to participate in capital punishment, or whether it is ethical to form a binding contract to serve as a surrogate mother. There is no legitimate grounds on which a professional organization, merely by being a professional organization, can claim authority on these matters. Given the eclectic makeup of professional organizations, inevitably one view or another will come to represent a plurality position—perhaps even a majority position—but that is no reason to assume that it therefore represents the position that must be adopted by all members of the profession. There is nothing inherent in being socialized into a profession that gives members, individually or collectively, claims to expertise on the moral norms related to the professional role. There is particularly no claim to expertise on the moral norms that bind the interaction with the patient, who is just as capable of reflecting on the moral norms for that interaction. Professionally generated moral norms simply fail to have the legitimacy that members of a religious or philosophical group attribute to their groups' theories of morality.

Conclusion

These three examples of the ways in which professional organizations articulate moral positions for medical professionals and laypeople serve only as illustrations. The examples could be repeated endlessly. These professional sources clearly are not the only possible sources of such norms for various professional and related lay roles. Religious and secular ethics present reasonable alternatives for laypeople who, in principle, cannot have the knowledge available only to the elite who have been brought into the wisdom of the professional group. Religious and secular ethics present reasonable alternatives even for the members of the profession who have the humility to recognize that they have no special moral knowledge comparable to their admitted technical expertise. In chapter 5 I turn to religious alternatives and then, in chapter 6, I consider secular alternatives.

CHAPTER

5

RELIGIOUS MEDICAL ETHICS

Revealed and Natural Alternatives

I F HIPPOCRATIC and other professionally generated codes of medical ethics fail to provide an adequate moral foundation for physicians who are not Pythagoreans—that is, for physicians who are simultaneously members of some non-Hippocratic religious or secular community with a worldview expressing a moral perspective—then the two obvious alternatives for professionals to get their ethics from are either religious or secular ethical systems. Here I consider religious sources of medical morality; I address secular sources in chapter 6.

Religiously committed physicians are in something of a bind if they accept the claim of the Hippocratic and other professional medical ethical traditions that the profession is responsible for generating or at least articulating the ethics for the profession. The religiously committed, after all, also profess loyalty to another system of belief and value that also purports to be the metaethical channel through with ethical norms are articulated. By nature, religion claims to affirm a relationship with a deity, and that deity is supposed to be the ground of being, including the ground of ethical obligation.

The ethical obligations that grow out of the various religious traditions claim to be inclusive. Their norms are norms for all of human conduct—including the conduct of professionals of all professions. Hence, a religiously committed member of a profession should reasonably look not to his or her professional group—made up of members who are committed to all manner of religious and secular belief systems—for moral authority. They should reasonably look to their religious groups for their norms—Talmudic ethics for Jewish physicians, Methodist ethics for Methodist physicians, Catholic ethics for Catholic physicians, and so on. Of course, sophisticated, religiously grounded ethics will incorporate norms for professionals when they are dealing with clients who do not share the practitioner's beliefs, but in any case, the norms would plausibly have their roots in the metaethical systems of the professional's religious tradition. Those norms would derive from the tradition's understanding of the origin or grounding of ethical obligation. The authoritative ways of knowing—the moral epistemology—would be the moral epistemology of the religious tradition; the authoritative texts, the texts of the religious tradition.

Thus we would expect a seriously Roman Catholic physician to accept some version of Catholic natural law doctrine, the belief that morality is part of the deity's created order, and the position that scripture and Church tradition, the Popes and Church councils, are authoritative. A seriously Lutheran physician who swore by Apollo rather than Yahweh and quoted Hippocrates rather than Luther would be confused—indeed, suspect. And it would not be any better for that Lutheran physician to cite modern professional medical ethical sources such as the Declaration of Geneva or the American Medical Association (AMA).

Religions claim that they have mechanisms of knowing divine truth or divine will. The claim almost always includes a comprehensive ethical system by means of which adherents know what is morally required of them. They may gain this knowledge through revelation or similar non-natural means of knowing, or may gain it through more straightforward affirmation of the role of reason, experience, or natural law (which in some cases may be seen as modes of revelation). They produce a branch of theology called theological ethics, and their ethic is comprehensive in the sense that it purports to explicate ethical norms for all branches of human endeavor, including the practice of the professions.

Hence, if one is a Catholic physician, one would expect to practice medicine following the teachings of the Church fathers. In contrast, the claim of the fathers of medicine to be a source of moral norms is anemic. No logic compels us to accept the idea that expertise in medical science, no matter how great, will also imply expertise in the moral norms relevant to the application of that science.

In the United States a Catholic physician seeking moral guidance would not plausibly turn to an ancient Greek oath of a Pythagorean-like mystery religion; she would turn to the "Ethical and Religious Directives for Catholic Health Facilities," the authoritative pronouncements of the Vatican including such statements as the "Declaration on Euthanasia," the birth control encyclical, *Humanae vitae*, and the Pontifical Academy for Life's statement on the use of embryonic stem cells, "Declaration on the Production and the Scientific and Therapeutic Use of Human Embryonic Stem Cells."[1] These pronouncements make use of sources, methods, and concepts appropriate for the group. None of these make moral sense for the secular physician or patient; they may call for secular concurrence, but they normally do not compel adherence. The theory of authority captured in these documents is consistent with the tradition to which these documents speak. Authorities are theological scholars, canon lawyers, and relevant teaching authorities of the Church. A physician or medical group would be seen as authoritative only to the extent that the physician or group could qualify in the hierarchy of ecclesiastical expertise. Conversely, a medical-ethical document generated outside that hierarchy of expertise would have little claim to epistemological status except insofar as Catholic natural law doctrine recognized the power of the reason or the thinking underlying such non-Catholic documents.

Of course, the individual who is generally identified with a particular religious tradition will not normally accept all its positions unthinkingly. Even relatively authoritarian traditions recognize the role of individual conscience. More egalitarian ones, such as Protestant traditions that affirm the "priesthood of all believers," give considerable authority to their lay members to interpret scripture and tradition. Nevertheless, the individual layperson who accepts membership in or identification with a religious tradition—even the individual layperson who is a health professional—will be inclined to accept the ways of knowing and sources of authority within that tradition, at least to a substantial degree. Otherwise, what is the meaning of identifying with the tradition?

The issue that must be confronted is whether professionally articulated codifications produced by the professional collectivity made up of a hodgepodge of practitioners with various secular and religious commitments can make a legitimate claim on the physician committed, at least predominantly, to one particular religious group. Of course, there are some base points of similarity in virtually all ethics. No religious code of ethics that I know comes out in favor of physicians having sexual relations with patients when they visit the patient's home. Similarly, benefiting the patient when there are no reasons against producing benefit would be hard for any religious or secular ethic to oppose. The morally interesting cases, however, are the ones for which reasons do exist for refraining from benefiting, at least from benefiting as the Hippocratic Oath would have the physician act—according to the physician's own judgment.

In some cases, benefit comes at the expense of doing great harm. The nineteenth-century "primum non nocere" slogan apparently would constrain patient benefit in that case. In some cases, benefit comes at the expense of violating patients' rights. The late-twentieth-century Patient's Bill of Rights, as well as most codes of the twenty-first century, would constrain patient benefit if it came at the expense of violating patients' rights. Hence, physicians should not benefit in Hippocratic fashion when it requires breaching confidentiality, failing to get consent, or lying to patients. In some cases, benefit to the patient comes at the expense of failing to do great good to others in society. All codes of ethics—religious, secular, and professional—since the days of ethical traditions contemporaneous to the Hippocratic text would require suppressing patient benefit if necessary to protect the society in certain cases of public health. In some cases, benefit to the patient comes at the expense of violating the principle of justice. Jewish, Christian, and most other religious codes of ethics will occasionally require the physician to refrain from benefiting the patient if patient benefit will produce great injustice to others, for example, if resources needed to benefit other worse-off patients will be squandered in producing very marginal benefits for an already well-off patient. In short, there are many moral requirements captured in religious ethical systems that are simply incompatible with Hippocratic and similar professional ethics oriented to patient benefit.

Revealed Religious Truths: An Alternative to Hippocratic Revelation

Some religious systems of ethics depend on nonnatural means of revelation of religious truths, including moral truths. Revealed truths in the various religions are direct competitors to the moral knowledge captured in Hippocratic and other professional oaths that claim that their knowledge is generated by the professional group itself or is knowable only by members of the group. Thus, the Hippocratic Oath's claim that knowledge of the group is esoteric, potent, and secret leads to the historical claim that only members of the group can know what is morally required for its members. These claims, however, are directly in conflict with similar claims made by advocates for religious traditions that believe in religious revelation of moral truths.

The Oath itself made such a claim. The knowledge of the Hippocratic group was secret and unknowable to those outside the group. Similarly, the Kappa Lambda Society of Hippocrates, a prominent early-nineteenth-century association of elite physicians that claimed Hippocrates as "the remote founder of this Society" and with chapters in a number of American cities, administered an oath that was also secret.[2] In fact, the entire organization was secret. Its very existence was kept from the general public and even from lesser physicians who were not invited to join.[3]

Historically, medical professional organizations have claimed that they not only have the responsibility for generating or articulating their code of ethics, they also claim that the code is secret and cannot be understood by medical laypeople. In 1970, when a physician from Manchester, England was accused of violating the promise of confidentiality and was tried before the General Medical Council of Great Britain, I contacted the British Medical Association to ask for a copy of its current code of ethics in order to understand the claim in this doctor's defense that his disclosure of patient medical information was consistent with the BMA code of the time. I was told by the BMA that their code of ethics was secret and could not be disclosed to nonmembers.

Although the AMA does not claim secrecy for its activities that attempt to govern the ethical conduct of physicians, it has, from its earliest days in 1847 until today, involved only its members on the committees and councils that promulgate its ethics. With the exception of a representative of the medical student association, all the members of AMA's Council on Ethical and Judicial Affairs, the body responsible for formulating and supervising the conduct of physicians in relation to patients, are physicians from the AMA membership.

In comparison, religious groups affirming revealed sources of knowledge pass by medical professional groups like ships in the night. These proponents of religious sources of revealed moral truths make precisely parallel claims to those made by professional groups that insist they have special access to esoteric knowledge not knowable through natural means. The only difference between professional organizations that claim to generate codes of ethics for their members and religious groups is that the professional organizations exclude laypeople from membership while the religious groups accept both professionals and laypeople. In the latter case, however, members of various professional groups would not normally possess special authority when it comes to knowing the revealed truths of the religion. A physician member of a mystical religious sect would have the status of a mere lay member of the group, positioned to learn from the spiritual leader who claims to be the channel of revelation.

Karl Barth

Karl Barth addressed knowledge of moral requiredness explicitly in his 1937–38 Gifford Lectures in Aberdeen. This is a plausible place to begin our examination from the perspective of one committed to the central importance of revelation for knowledge of God.[4]

Barth's Defense of His Lectures: "Partner in the Conversation"

Barth was a strange and controversial choice to give the Gifford Lectures, and he knew it. The Giffords are supposed to be dedicated to "promoting, advancing, teaching, and diffusing the study of natural theology in the widest sense of that term."[5] Karl Barth is perhaps the single most militant opponent of natural theology since Martin Luther. The invitation was calculated to produce a clash.

Barth was well aware of this, and he began his lectures somewhat apologetically explaining why he could not do justice to the task in "direct agreement" with Lord Gifford's wishes:

> A reformed theologian commissioned with the delivery of these lectures cannot, as such, i.e., in loyalty towards his own calling, be in a position to do justice to this task in direct agreement and fulfilment of the intention of the testator. He can, however, make this task his own indirectly. He can, namely, confer on "natural theology" the loyal and real service of reminding it of its partner in the conversation. If it wishes to achieve its end in the sense used by the testator it has at least to enter into controversy with this partner, in opposition to whom it must make itself known, prove itself and maintain itself as truth if it is the truth![6]

For Barth the task Lord Gifford had in mind of advancing the science by which humans have natural knowledge of God unaided by revelation is simply an impossibility. Speaking of natural theology, he says: "I do not see how it is possible for it to exist. I am convinced that so far as it has existed and still exists, it owes its existence to a radical error."[7]

Barth then goes on to describe the "partner in the conversation"—that is, the opposition to natural theology to which Barth claims the Protestant reformation must be committed: "The positive content of the Reformation is the renewal of the church, based upon the revelation of God in Jesus Christ and this means implicitly the negation of all 'natural theology.' And 'natural theology' can only be developed in implicit and explicit negation of the Reformed teaching."[8] Barth, in short, will devote his Gifford Lectures on natural theology to defending his view on revelation as the source of all religious knowledge and correlatively the "negation" of all natural theology.

All Theological Knowledge Is Revealed and Not Natural   For Barth, the starting point of a medical morality must be religious knowledge—what he calls "faith knowledge"—known exclusively through revelation: "Faith knowledge is knowledge through revelation. And that simply means that it is a type of knowledge which is unconditionally bound to its object. And it is only to this object, only to God, that human thought can be bound in this way, since God Himself has bound it to Himself."[9] This revelation is, according to Barth, first and foremost through Jesus Christ, the central figure of all Christian religious groups, but particularly crucial for Barth and the Reformed Church: "Knowledge of God, according to the teaching of the Reformation, consists, as we have seen, in the knowledge of the God who deals with man in His Revelation in Jesus Christ. Knowledge of God according to the teaching of the Reformation does not therefore permit the man who knows to withdraw himself from God, so to speak, and to maintain an independent and secure position over against God so that from this he may form thoughts about God, which are in varying degrees true, beautiful and good."[10]

Barth then immediately goes on to argue that this latter way of knowing from an "independent and secure position over against God" is the focus of the larger Gifford project and what Barth must reject. There can be no independent, objective knowledge apart from revelation. For Barth, "it is not a matter here of observing, analysing, considering and judging an object, where the knower is permitted to consider himself disinterested, free and superior in his relation to his object."[11] This latter procedure, says Barth,

> is that of all natural theology. One can only choose between this and the procedure of Reformed theology, one cannot reconcile them. Knowledge of God according to the teaching of the Reformation is obedience to God and therefore itself already service of God. According to Reformed teaching the knowledge of God is brought about when the object reaches out and grasps the subject, and through this the latter, the man who knows, becomes a new man. All thoughts which he forms about God can only be an echo of what was said to him through God's dealing with him, by means of which he became this new man.[12]

Knowledge of Ethics Is Theological Knowledge Available Only through Revelation   For our purposes, the critical issue is how this is relevant to Barth's theory of knowledge in ethics, especially medical ethics. In his massive (originally two-volume) 1928 work titled *Ethics*, Barth devotes his first sections to an explication of the relation of his ethics to his dogmatics, that is, his systematic theology, and then his views on the relation of theological ethics to philosophical ethics.[13] It quickly becomes clear how forcefully he rejects not only natural theology but also any anthropocentric ethics including any philosophical foundation for ethics.

For him, the absolutely necessary starting point of dogmatics is revelation, "the Word revealed in scripture."[14] He regards any methodological distinction between ethics and dogmatics as "ethically suspect."[15] This is because separation involves a change in focus from God to man, which in turn rests on "the suspicious hypothesis that revelation puts theology in a position to speak of God and man in one and the same breath."[16]

In the second section he takes up the relation of theological ethics and philosophical ethics. He acknowledges that "ethics is not originally or self-evidently theological ethics."[17] Philosophical ethics has its grounding in human history, which leaves the philosophical ethicist with the problem of finding a standard or a foundation for judging human conduct. When the philosopher strays into the realm of theological ethics, he finds himself "in a strange world," a place where knowledge comes from sources that are incomprehensible and alien to him.[18] This, says Barth, is no problem at all for the theologian. For the Barthian theologian doing ethics, his starting point is "the concept of the reality of the God who has dealings with man through his Word . . . the inwardly secure and presupposed starting point of every question and answer."[19] Thus, for Barth, ethics done theologically is necessarily theological knowledge. It is gained through the revealed Word—that is, scripture.

Examples of Barth's Ethics Applied to Medicine   Barth does not devote a great deal of attention to the applications of his theological method relating revelation to ethical norms for human conduct. He is especially stingy in spelling out his positions on medical ethical issues. His approach, however, is quite clear. At various places he takes up topics central to medicine: respect for life and euthanasia, abortion, contraceptives, and the role of the doctor, for example. His starting point in each case is scripture—the revealed Word of God.

Respect for Life/Euthanasia. In *Church Dogmatics*, III/4, Barth takes up the topic of respect for life.[20] He launches the discussion by attacking an earlier Gifford lecturer, Albert Schweitzer, who had addressed the topic of the problem of natural theology and natural ethics in 1934 and 1935. The lectures, unfortunately, were never published. Barth focuses his attack on Schweitzer's philosophy of civilization (*Kultur und Ethik*). He zeros in on Schweitzer's claim that life—our own life and that of others—is the supreme good. Barth dissents: "It goes without saying that theological ethics cannot accept this."[21] To Barth, this is a rejection of the divine authority. "Where Schweitzer places life we see the command of God."[22] Says Barth, "Man is . . . commanded to live."[23] Thus, for Barth, his pro-life ethics is not a recognition of the preciousness of human life per se but more a response to the divine command made known to man through revelation transmitted in the scriptures.

Barth goes on to build a consistent respect-for-life ethic claiming that

> life does not itself create this respect. The command of God creates respect for it. When man in faith in God's Word and promise realises how God from eternity has maintained and loved him in his little life, and what He had done for him in time, in this knowledge of human life he is faced by a majestic, dignified and holy fact. In human life itself he meets something superior. He is thus summoned to respect because the living God has distinguished it in this way and taken it to Himself. We may confidently say that the birth of Jesus Christ as such is the revelation of the command as that of respect for life.[24]

The issue for us here is not to understand Barth's claim or how he knows the truth of what he takes to be revealed in what he calls the "Word"; it is to see that his bioethics gets its momentum from what he takes to be knowledge by way of revelation. He looks with disdain on Schweitzer's more natural ways of knowing.

Abortion. Barth's pro-life bioethics carries over to his views on abortion. He is, in fact, more militantly pro-life, if possible, than the Roman Catholic Church. Abortion is "irrefutably seen to be sin, murder, and transgression."[25] His is not the natural law argument on abortion of the Roman Catholic Church that its theologians claim can be known by reasoning human beings. His is a "No" to abortion known more surely to him than what is known by man's fallible reason. He asks "how this No is to be established and stated if it is to be truly effective."[26] His answer is it is not known by "mere churchmanship, whether Romanist or Protestant." Rather it is the "command of God . . . based on His grace."[27] Thus, it is not merely the word of man but the Word of God, known through revelation in the scriptures.

Contraception. Barth devotes several pages in *Church Dogmatics* III/4 to the extended struggle within his own mind over the ethics of birth control, a topic at the time of its writing that was a much more vivid controversy than it is today. He wrestles with arguments that the use of birth control may be either in accord with divine law or "something which the divine law strictly forbids."[28] In this ambiguity he stakes out a very cautious opening to contraception that is consistent with the writings of other Protestant figures at the time.[29]

Barth attempts to sharply differentiate his position from the Roman Catholic not only in his openness to birth control decisions but also on the grounds of his reasoning. He makes clear he is rejecting teleological appeals to natural law functions of marriage and the human body. He moves instead to the task of attempting to determine the "rule of divine providence." He writes: "For surely the providence of God and the course of nature are not identical or even on the same level. Surely the former cannot be inferred from the latter! Surely the providence and will of God in the course of nature has in each case to be freshly discovered by the believer who hears and obeys His word, and apprehended and put into operation by him in personal responsibility, in the freedom of choice and decision."[30] Here the individual conscience must be formed by access to the divine will apprehended by access to scriptural sources, not by argument over the natural functions or by the use of natural law—a rather explicit reference to Barth's rejection of Catholic medical morality.

The Role of the Physician. One last example of Barth's theocentric analysis of medical roles will reveal the complex dynamic of his views. He takes up what he refers to as "the will to be healthy" and the role of the physician in carrying out that will.[31] Having already argued that humans are subject to the divine command to have respect for life, he now claims that this respect for life includes the will to be healthy. This permits him to provide a discourse on the human's pursuit of health and the role of the physician in that pursuit. He considers the possibility that an individual's health and sickness is a subjective thing and that, therefore, the physician, as a relative stranger to this subjectivity, cannot know much about an individual's strength or weakness.[32] He ends up concluding that this is mistaken, that the physician can at least have expertise in the "psychical and physical functions."[33]

What is critical, however, is Barth's unusual and obscure notion of health that he feels humans should be inclined to will. He repeats several times in this section the odd phrase that "health is the strength to be as man."[34] It is clear that this notion of being "as man" has an overtly religious meaning for Barth. It requires man "not merely to be healthy in body and soul but to be man at all: man and not animal or plant, man and not wood or stone, man and not a thing or the exponent of an idea, man in the satisfaction of his instinctive needs, man in the use of his reason, in loyalty to his individuality, in the knowledge of its limitations, man in his relation to God and his fellow-men in the proffered act of freedom."[35]

This must surely be the most unique, convoluted, and theologically embedded notion of the concept of health in the history of medicine. It makes clear that Barth's understanding of the "psychical and physical" functions for which the human should turn to the physician are carefully linked to Barth's theological anthropology, his understanding of the human's status as a creature of the deity subject to the divine command. As such, it is not surprising that Barth claims that physicians can perform the function of promoting "strength to be as man" if (presumably, only if) they are "Christian doctors."[36] Without knowledge of God revealed in the Word of God, the physician is powerless to know how to facilitate the psychological and physical functions necessary for promoting the human's "strength to be as man."

The Isolation of Revealed Ethics Barth is certainly right when he says that the secular person would find himself "in a strange world" upon hearing this account of how one knows what is morally required of a medical practitioner. It is not too much to say that, from the perspective of a nonbeliever, this is pure nonsense. Fortunately, for our purposes, we do not have to pass judgment on whether Barth's moral epistemology relying on divine command revealed in the scriptures is defensible.

My project is to understand the implications of such a view for professionally generated and articulated medical ethics—the ethics of the Hippocratic Oath, the World Medical Association's Declaration of Geneva, or the AMA's Principles of Medical Ethics. Quite obviously for the Barthian physician or patient who relied on Barth's claims about knowledge of God through revelation, including moral knowledge of God's commands, the professionally generated codifications are utterly without standing. They make absolutely no use of the knowledge that, for Barth, is crucial.

This has radical implications for religious believers who want medicine practiced morally from their point of view. In some parts of the world, including some parts of the United States, it is not uncommon for physicians to simultaneously be devout members of fundamentalist, evangelical, or other confessional Christian churches. Some of these accept more or less Barthian notions that reject natural knowledge of morality in favor of moral knowledge revealed by the divinity through scripture or, as we shall see shortly, by more direct mystical communication with certain believers. The physician who wants to practice medicine morally and who believes that morality has its foundation in divine command revealed through scripture should have no use for the AMA's Council on Ethical and Judicial Affairs. Such physicians rely on a much higher authority.

More critically, patients who are members of such religious groups that rely on Barthian notions of revealed epistemology would be wise to guard against engaging physicians who lack these sources of revelation. How could the believing patient trust a physician with critical matters of life and death, procreation and mental health, if that physician relied on a source of moral norms so alien to that patient's professed belief that all human morality is response to divine command revealed through religious sources such as scripture and church tradition? It would be not only irrational but truly dangerous to place one's life and health in the hands of a physician, no matter how skilled, if that physician made no pretense of having access to such crucial moral knowledge and, if, in fact, he or she professed loyalty to external sources of medical morality articulated by a nonbelieving, secular group of mere professionals. From the point of view of the Barthian patient, a moral medical professional would have to be one who had some degree of access to the truth as revealed. From the point of view of the Barthian physician, the only legitimate way to practice medicine would be from within the perspective of the faith tradition that had special access to revealed moral truth.

Presumably, there is not much outsiders could do to encourage medical morality for such believers. They should be left on their own. As long as they are in patient-physician pairs that share the same faith in their moral epistemologies, and as long as innocent, unconsenting parties are not harmed, there may be no reason to interfere. This could mean that, from the outsider's point of view, great tragedy results. Jehovah's Witness adults may die from lack of blood transfusions; Christian Scientist patients may die refusing penicillin and preferring instead to seek counsel of Christian Science practitioners. More controversially, it may mean that women with life-threatening pregnancies or those carrying fetuses with painful terminal conditions will carry their pregnancies to term with the aid and support of their similarly inclined medical practitioners. From an outsider's point of view, these may be tragic outcomes, but it is probably the price that a society pays for a robust belief in the freedom of people to make their own religious commitments and live by them as long as innocent third parties are not harmed. It seems clear, however, that such patients and such physicians will find little worthwhile in the articulated medical ethical guidance of medical professional groups. It would be irrational for a Barthian patient or a Barthian physician to rely on such sources of moral guidance.

Stanley Hauerwas

Although Barth comments very sparingly on matters of medical ethics, a more recent Gifford lecturer who stands in the Barthian tradition is much more committed to bioethics. Stanley Hauerwas, the Gilbert T. Rowe Professor of Theological Ethics at Duke University's Divinity School, gave the Giffords in 2001 at the University of St. Andrews. The lectures were published as *With the Grain of the Universe: The Church's Witness and Natural Theology*.[37] Hauerwas is probably the only Gifford lecturer other than Barth to respond to Lord Gifford's mandate to study natural theology by boldly attacking it in the name of revealed theology.[38]

Hauerwas takes on the works of three previous Gifford lecturers—Barth, William James, and Reinhold Niebuhr—and claims that Niebuhr (one of the other of the pantheon of famed mid-twentieth-century theologians widely seen as attacking theological liberalism) falls into the trap of natural theology in a way reminiscent of James's more overtly secular reliance on attempts to be objective and scientific in an account of religion.

Hauerwas's Reconstruction of Natural Theology   Hauerwas's core argument is that, of the three previous lecturers that Hauerwas reviews, only Barth survives as "the great natural theologian of the Gifford Lectures—at least he is so if you remember that natural theology is the attempt to witness to the nongodforsakenness of the world even under the conditions of sin."[39] Herein lies a subtle difference between Hauerwas and Barth. Barth affirms revelation as the sole source of knowledge of God (and therefore God's command that becomes the legitimate grounding of theological ethics), thereby rejecting natural theology and natural knowledge of morality's norms. Hauerwas, on the other hand, while sharing Barth's reliance on revelation of the deity, ends up claiming that the knowledge of the world that is known through revelation in fact becomes the legitimate grounds for knowing about nature (including about the nature of morality). Hauerwas reconstructs the meaning of natural theology so that Barth becomes "the great natural theologian of the Gifford Lectures."[40]

This, I suggest, is something of a linguistic trick—making the modern world's most hostile critic of natural ways of knowing about theology and ethics into its most reliable proponent of the newly minted natural theology. For Hauerwas, it is only through revelation that we gain true knowledge of the world, including the world of ethics; therefore, he feels entitled to call Barth's work (and his own) "natural theology." This, of course, misses the point of Lord Gifford and others of us who are striving mightily to bridge those working in religious ethics and those compelled to more secular, nontheistic approaches to ethics. It fails in addressing the core problem of whether nonbelievers and believers can have enough moral knowledge in common to develop a medical ethic suitable for a more universal foundation of the practice of medicine between medical professionals, who may have only the most rudimentary interest in and knowledge of theology, and medical laypeople, whose moral worldview is shaped by a set of fundamental religious (or philosophical) commitments. If true "natural theology" is, as Hauerwas suggests, grounded in a wholly otherworldly confession of the divine command knowable only by nonnatural means, then calling the resulting knowledge of the moral world "natural" seems to be something of theological sleight of hand.

Hauerwas's Reliance on Revealed Morality in His Medical Ethics

In contrast to Barth, Hauerwas writes widely on matters of medical ethics. However, he is not as explicit as Barth in stating how he believes one gains knowledge of moral requiredness. Given his Barthian sympathies and his extensive comments on matters of medical morality, it seems clear that he relies on unique religious sources in ways similar to Barth.

In his *Suffering Presence: Theological Reflection on Medicine, the Mentally Handicapped, and the Church*, Hauerwas comes closer to stating his position than in most of his other writings. His chapter "Salvation and Health: Why Medicine Needs the Church" provides some insights into his views on the foundation of medical morality. Here he claims Christian ethics is different from other kinds of ethics.[41] In Barthian fashion, he bemoans those doing Christian ethics without any sense of distinctive commitments as theologians.[42] He notes that his mentor complains that modern philosophy has not been able to provide a persuasive account of moral obligation.[43] The task of theologians, says Hauerwas, is to supply the needed rationale. Pointing to his earlier treatment of preservation of life in his *Vision and Virtue*, he claims that Christians do not share the same attitudes as non-Christians. He even suggests that it makes sense to think of a "Christian medicine."[44] If moral norms of the sort that he considers relevant are knowable only through revelation of the divine command, then those with access to that special knowledge would practice medicine differently in the sense that their objectives, including the decisions rendered when it comes to preserving life, will be radically different and incomprehensible to outsiders (including the outsiders at the center or organized medicine's articulation of its norms).

In his theological reflection on in vitro fertilization, Hauerwas makes clear that he is speaking from this special theological perspective that provides special knowledge. "I do not pretend to speak from principles that are or should be shared by everyone in our society."[45] This means that, for Hauerwas, any presumption of "moral agreement or consensus among many philosophical and religious ethicists is unfounded."[46] When moral knowledge has its foundation in divine command knowable only as revealed truth, any such agreement would have no basis. Thus, a radically different medicine, a Christian medicine, would be called for. Professional sources, uninformed by this unique source of moral knowledge, would be vacuous.

Oral Roberts

An even more fascinating example of a Protestant who builds a medical ethic from revealed sources of moral knowledge is the American evangelical Oral Roberts.[47] His approach to knowledge of what is required in medical ethics shares with Barth and Hauerwas the key characteristic of reliance on specialized nonnatural knowledge and can be summarized more briefly.

Long committed to the evangelical bedrock premise of the inerrancy of scripture as the revealed truth of the divine power, Roberts also claimed direct revelation to him from the deity. He followed his premises to their logical conclusion. From his point of view it should be impossible to know what is ethically required in the practice of medicine without direct access to scripture or other special revelation. Physicians practicing medicine without such guidance would be sailing blind. It should be impossible.

Roberts created an evangelically based health care system with patients and health professionals recruited because they shared his views about the foundation of medical morality in scriptural revelation. Central to his vision, for example, was the assigning of a "prayer partner" to each patient. Physicians would explicitly incorporate prayer into their healing. He built the $250 million City of Faith Medical Center in which the Oral Roberts brand of health care could be delivered, presumably with the mutual consent of all parties involved. His Oral Roberts University included a medical school so physicians could be educated into the proper perspective for the practice of medicine. These parties shared the belief that moral choices about health care—about abortion, euthanasia, and out-of-wedlock in vitro fertilization—could only be made with scriptural or other revealed guidance. For those who share this fundamental metaethic of revelation, it would surely be irrational to draw on the Hippocratic ethic as made known in a pagan, Pythagorean-like Greek mystery religion. Thus, religious ethics grounded in revelation once again must offer a medical ethic completely independent of, and often at odds with, Hippocratic ethics or its more recent professionally generated counterparts. Only by coincidence could the esoteric knowledge known only to the Pythagoreans converge with the esoteric knowledge known to Oral Roberts.

The Lutheran Tradition

Although the views about natural law in the tradition of Martin Luther are complex, Lutheran commentators have generally followed Martin Luther in doubting the role of a natural law, including its role in generating moral norms for the practice of medicine.[48] Hence, seriously committed Lutheran patients and Lutheran health professionals may be forced into a position similar to that of Barth and Roberts. They may know, by faith, certain moral norms that cannot be explained by reason. Even though these norms are seen as shaping the way medicine should be practiced, it is difficult to imagine how those outside of the faith would have any understanding.

Thus, Lutheran health providers may be forced into positions in which they believe they know through their religious sources of moral knowledge the correct medical decisions to make when caring for patients, but they are at a loss to explain them to nonbelievers except by stating they know what is revealed to them in scripture. Likewise, Lutheran patients should find objectionable receipt of medical care from a provider outside their own tradition who could not possibly be expected to have the benefit of revealed moral truths.

For example, one of the primary tenets of Lutheran thought is a robust belief in human finitude that leaves all condemned to acknowledge the probability of moral error. At the same time, though fallible, even the layperson is capable, to some degree, of reading and interpreting scripture. There is, to use the standard term, a "priesthood of all believers." Hence, one might expect a truly Lutheran hospital to have a medical records department that looks radically different from a Hippocratic one.

The Hippocratic tradition believed that knowledge of the patient's condition was often best kept in the hands of the professional. The Pythagorean-like system believed that such information was potent and could cause trouble in the hands of the uninitiated. In modern times, Hippocratic practitioners often believed that disclosing a diagnosis or even a medication name to a patient was often considered too dangerous. Patients as late as the 1960s were routinely not told of a terminal diagnosis.[49] Information about diagnosis was to be dispensed, like potent medicine, only when "indicated." It was normally to be withheld from laypeople who could be upset or injured if they received the unvarnished truth.[50]

By contrast, one would expect a Lutheran hospital's physicians and its medical records department to behave much differently, at least if it took Lutheran theology and its related epistemology seriously. If the central teaching of the church is that the layperson can be trusted to have access to and to interpret the text, then, in medicine, that surely must mean that normally they should have access to their own medical records. A policy of routine access to hospital charts and the advice necessary to help understand them is plausibly the only way Lutherans could run a medical records department. There is no quantum difference in capacity to understand between the priest initiated into the mysteries of the practice and the layperson given reasonable orientation. Names of diagnoses and of medications are now, in a post-Hippocratic era, routinely given to patients. It is widely believed that patients are better off if they are educated about their conditions and the medications they are taking. That is the medical equivalent of the Lutheran doctrine of the priesthood of all believers.

Even though all humans are fallible and subject to the risk of erroneous interpretation of the text, the medical layperson is no more fallible than the medical professional in this regard. If theological laypersons can be trusted with the scriptural texts, then medical laypersons surely can be trusted with the medical texts.

Judaism

A fifth and more complex example of a religious ethic that has the potential to provide a foundation for medical morality is Judaism. It can be argued that Yahweh's revelation of the Decalogue to Moses was also a special revealed source of moral knowledge available and applicable only to those who are part of the group. That Decalogue provides, in brief, moral content believed to be the divine law, which guides believers in their secular practices, including the practice of medicine. Knowledge about the morality of lying to patients, killing, adultery, and organ transplant can all be gleaned from commentary on the Decalogue and the remainder of the Pentateuch. More esoteric dietary law, requirements about circumcision, autopsy, the burial of the dead, and physician travel on the Sabbath are all ferreted out of these texts by rabbinical scholars. At least some of these Talmudic laws are incomprehensible to Gentiles and others who deny the authority of the texts.

For example, the ethics of procuring organs for transplant poses something of a dilemma for the rabbinical scholar who knows that the corpse should not be desecrated but that saving the life of another is an even higher moral responsibility.[51] This is not an issue for the Gentile for whom religious law pertaining to handling of the corpse is not an issue. Any Jewish scholar will tell us that this apparent dilemma has an easy solution for the Jew—an exception is made to the normal prohibition on desecration of the dead when procuring a life-saving organ such as a heart or a liver is at stake. Furthermore, most rabbis will tell us that even organs and tissues that are less immediately connected with life-saving, such as kidneys and corneas, may be procured in the name of saving life. It is argued that the sighted man stands a better chance of avoiding death by accident than one who is blind, and that cornea transplants are, in the end, life saving.

Judaism, however, offers more than the Mosaic covenant. The earlier covenants offer moral norms that apply to all humans, Gentile as well as Jew. They are knowable not only through revelation but also through knowledge of the natural order—through human reason or experience. Thus, Judaism can be said to offer us a two-tiered way of having moral knowledge—through natural processes available to all and through more specific, supernatural divine intervention such as the revelation to Moses on Mt. Sinai. This two-tiered moral epistemology offers promise for how we might understand medical morality in a post-Hippocratic age.

The Complex Case of Tristram Engelhardt

A vivid example of this two-tiered moral epistemology for the ethics of medicine is seen in the works of Orthodox Christian physician-philosopher H. Tristram Engelhardt. His earlier writings focused mainly on what one could know in a secular, pluralistic world about the ethical foundations of bioethics. His starting point was a search for what could be known by humans that would generate agreement as an alternative to the use of force.[52] The product was a very thin ethic resting on the principle of autonomy (called the principle of permission in his later edition) that permitted interference with the freedom of others only with their permission.[53] For the secular Engelhardt, that was all that reason required (provided one was committed to eschewing the use of force). The result was a libertarian ethic envisioning many different practices of medicine among mutually agreeing health professionals and patients.

There is, however, another side to Engelhardt, especially in his later years. Since his conversion to Orthodoxy he has also written about Christian bioethics.[54] The result is a much richer, thicker ethic for the patient–

physician relation among those who share the commitment to Engelhardt's version of Christianity. For Engelhardt, a radically different moral epistemology is inherent in Christian bioethics. It concedes the failure of rational discourse as a basis for establishing what he calls a "content-full" ethic. Hence, he rejects natural law approaches of Roman Catholic moral theologians.[55] The traditional secular ways of relying on reason and experience are unsuccessful in bringing about a common set of moral principles upon which a medical ethic can be based. While Engelhardt does not use the language of Barth and Hauerwas of revealed moral truth, he advocates reliance on a different kind of knowing that he identifies with Orthodox, traditional Christianity—the ways of knowing that predate the Renaissance, Reformation, and Enlightenment, a position closely connected with his conversion to Orthodoxy.[56]

This, for Engelhardt, involves a radically different way of knowing: "The moral epistemology underlying Christian bioethics is unlike that which can be claimed for secular bioethics. Or to put matters another way, the collapse of Christian bioethics into secular bioethics is only avoided when one recalls that the epistemological claims of Christian bioethics are rooted in a real experience of a transcendent God. In the absence of a noetic experience, religious knowledge will always only be immanent."[57]

In a manner reminiscent of Barth and Hauerwas but with a distinctly Orthodox character, Engelhardt puts forward what he calls a "noetic" way of knowing, knowing with the heart or knowledge coming from an immediate experience of the deity.[58] This noetic experience, says Engelhardt, "is the sufficient condition required to establish a Christian bioethics."[59] This makes clear why, for Engelhardt, moral knowledge for a medical ethic is fundamentally different from what is available in secular bioethics or its rationalist equivalent in natural theology. The project of natural law ethics of the Roman Catholic theologians is, in Engelhardt's view, doomed to fail.

Engelhardt uses the language of "natural law" in a way that is not altogether negative. In the spirit of Hauerwas and drawing on the traditional Orthodox writers St. John of Chrysostom and St. Isaac of Syria, he speaks of "natural knowledge" inherent in humans, but by this he means not our capacity to reason but our capacity to "know in our hearts what we ought to do."[60] Hence, Engelhardt can be added to the list of religious bioethicists who rely on special kinds of knowledge for the structuring of the moral relations between health professional and patient. He endorses a special bioethics that cannot be available to secular thinkers and those outside this special noetic way of knowing. Professionally generated ethical codifications for him—as for Barth, Hauerwas, Roberts, and those subject to the Mosaic covenant—are outside the bounds of moral insight.

The Implications of Religiously Revealed Ethics

While the religious systems that rely on revelation through scripture and direct communication from the deity differ radically among themselves, they all pose a similar problem. Physicians who accept a revealed religious epistemology for the grounding of their ethical knowledge should find professionally articulated ethics to be without authority—indeed, irrelevant. No matter how diverse, those who accept revealed sources, through scripture or direct divine communication, must believe that the moral codes articulated by the professional group of physicians, at least a professional agency outside their religious group, stand outside the authoritative pipeline of information.

Why would a physician who accepts Karl Barth's or Oral Roberts's understanding of moral knowledge give any weight to the moral code of a group that has no capacity to receive the revealed truth? A City of Faith doctor who accepts the claim of Oral Roberts that God speaks directly to him on moral and other matters surely should be unmoved by a diverse group of secular physicians who make up the AMA's Council on Ethical and Judicial Affairs and have the responsibility for drawing up the AMA's ethical code. They should have even less interest in codes of the professional organizations of other countries. From this point of view, the professional code writers are morally blind.

The health professional who adheres to a religious system that claims revealed sources of moral knowledge for leading daily life (including professional life) is, on the other hand, in a position similar to that of the physicians originally committed to the Hippocratic Oath. He has access to privileged communication that the patient who is outside the religious system cannot be expected to comprehend.

Consider, for example, the awkward position of the Christian Science practitioner. When caring for Christian Science patients, both practitioner and patient share a common set of epistemological beliefs. Those beliefs, however, are alien to those outside the Christian Science world who reject its moral (and medical) ontology. Christian Science practitioners should be at a loss to explain their moral and scientific beliefs to patients who are outside that belief system. They are structurally analogous to a Hippocratic physician who believes moral knowledge is transmitted only to those initiated into the Hippocratic school.

There is one critical difference, however, between medical professionals who accept a revealed religious source of moral knowledge and Hippocratic physicians. In the case of Barthian or City of Hope physicians, there is every reason to assume that they are in a community where they can practice medicine with like-minded medical laypeople who also accept the claims of their particular brand of revealed religion. On the other hand, ordinary laypeople who do not share the professional's religious worldview should fear a doctor who would practice medicine according to the revealed dictates of the believer in dialectical theology or mystical conversations between spiritual leader and deity. All manner of revealed moral oddities could directly impact the way medicine is practiced. The patient who is not part of the special religious community would be made victim of the revelation as perceived by the practitioner. By contrast, the layperson who shares the religious worldview of the practitioner should feel comfortable knowing that her doctor has access to what both patient and provider believe is the divine moral command. Presumably patients standing within those faith traditions should fear only the secular physician not privileged to have similar access to the divine word.

In this way, the medicine practiced by the believers in revealed morality differs critically from that of the Hippocratic physician. The Hippocratic physician was the beneficiary of revelation of secret knowledge through the Pythagorean-like mystery cult, knowledge so potent and dangerous that the initiate pledges not to reveal the secrets to ordinary laypeople. Thus, not only does the Hippocratic physician have privileged access to special knowledge about the moral requirements of the practice of medicine but also no laypeople—that is, no patients—can share in that knowledge. That same exclusivity is claimed in professionally generated ethics into modern times, whether Kappa Lambda's secret society of elite physicians in nineteenth-century America or the British Medical Association in 1970 when it claimed that its code of ethics was secret and not available to those outside the professional group. Thus, literally every patient who is not also a member of the Hippocratic cult or its modern equivalent and whose doctor accepts the Hippocratic epistemology of professionally revealed moral truths must be an outsider, one who does not have knowledge of these truths except through accepting the word of the initiate.

Barth and Roberts were both medical laypersons, no matter how rigorously they claimed access to divine revelation. Thus, if they received medical care from followers who happened to be physicians, they shared with those physicians common beliefs about the moral truths known through the special knowledge conveyed through their special sources. By contrast, no patient receiving health care from a Hippocratic provider who claims to be practicing medicine based on professionally articulated moral norms can claim a commonly shared capacity to know the moral premises of the provider's practice.

It is not that the Hippocratic and other professionally generated or articulated codes of ethics contain odd or controversial norms, although they surely do. The absence of any consent doctrine, the militant disinterest in the common good, and the oddly worded abortion prohibition all are grounds for concern, but that is not the real problem. The real problem is the metaethical claim that the professional group is solely responsible for its own code of ethics and claims an epistemically privileged position so that its members are the only ones capable of learning the moral norms that govern the professional–patient relation. When a religion claiming epistemically privileged access to revelation puts forward odd moral norms, it at least includes both professionals and laypeople among its adherents. It would impose those norms on outsiders only if its professionals used those norms to govern conduct with outsiders.

Whether religious groups that claim privileged sources of revealed knowledge of the moral law for lay–professional relations pose a threat to the broader, secular society will depend upon whether the special esoteric duties believed to be required by those who accept these special revelations impose additional duties that are incomprehensible to outsiders but compatible with secular moral norms or whether, alternatively, they impose special duties that conflict with the norms of the broader society. If all a group claiming special revelation imposes is an added level of duty, then the broader secular society need not feel distress. If, for example, Orthodox Jews feel compelled to follow special dietary law or to refuse abortion, the secular world should be able to tolerate these beliefs even if they are not understood by the outsider. If, however, the group that claims special revelation of norms affirms a set of duties that are perceived as conflicting with the norms of the broader secular society, then a potential conflict is likely.

For example, Jews who refuse autopsy may find themselves in conflict with secular norms that require autopsy for public health purposes. Christian Scientists who refuse orthodox medical treatments for their children may find themselves in conflict with secular norms that require reasonable medical care for the incompetent children in a family. A culture that practices female circumcision may find itself in conflict with secular norms that protect young women and girls from what appears to be inhumane practice.

The bottom line is that religious traditions that affirm special nonnatural sources of knowledge for their moral norms may be able to develop alternative medical practices that can function in parallel to mainstream medicine. If physicians who affirm association with religious groups that claim special sources of moral knowledge practice their medicine only on patients who share that perspective and do not violate norms considered critical by the broader society, little harm is likely to result. At least no rights are violated. The medical practitioners and their patients surely would have no reason to cede moral authority to a medical professional organization such as the AMA. Organized medicine with ethics in the hands of members who are not privileged with access to special revelation should have no basis for understanding the moral norms affirmed by members of these more sectarian traditions. What should result is a separate sectarian practice of medicine (what Hauerwas called "Christian medicine") that makes sense to medical professionals and patients alike who share the beliefs about special sources of knowledge. These will be incomprehensible to those outside of those belief systems, just as mainstream medicine and ethics are perceived by those inside these belief systems as inadequate.

Natural Theology and Religious Moral Knowledge

It is here that the other major way of gaining religious knowledge becomes critical. The moral epistemology of the religious traditions also includes, in some cases, acceptance of natural ways of knowing moral norms. If a practitioner of medicine is committed to a religious tradition that accepts these natural ways of knowing—what Lord Gifford would have thought of as natural theology as it applies to the realm of moral epistemology for religious people—then that practitioner in principle shares a common moral knowledge with patients who likewise accept natural ways of knowing morally.

Roman Catholic Medical Ethics

The most obvious and important example is the great tradition of Roman Catholic medical morality. Medical ethics for mainstream Roman Catholics is a subcategory of their natural law theory of ethics as articulated since the days of Thomas Aquinas.[61] Through an elaborate theoretical system, mainstream Catholic scholars have believed that God created natural laws that govern the creation and that the natural law is moral, for human existence (as opposed to inanimate, vegetative, or animal existence), in the sense that it is within human free will to conform to or reject the law. It is a teleological form of natural law theory according to which all entities are created with an end in mind. Discernment of these ends permits judgments about whether a particular action is in accord with those ends. Knowledge of these ends and the moral natural law associated with it is, in principle, knowable by reason.

Recent developments in Catholic natural law theory suggest that the scholastic tradition is still very much alive. Notre Dame theologian Jean Porter, for example, actively pursues a contemporary account reconstructing the theological natural law tradition for modern times.[62] She offers a revisiting of Aquinas and the scholastics, suggesting what she describes as "a way of thinking about the natural law that is distinctively theological, while at the same time remaining open to other intellectual perspectives, including those of the natural sciences."[63] She offers an explanation of the relation of the teleological account of natural law to ethical realism and natural rights.

Catholic natural law thinking has had robust implications for the practice of medicine. Obvious major positions have been staked out on such chestnuts as abortion, euthanasia, contraception, sterilization, and the use of stem cells.[64] What is less well known is that the moral tradition grounded in Catholic natural doctrine has sweeping implications for the day-to-day practice of medicine even in areas that are not as stereotypically ethical. The Catholic duty to prepare spiritually for one's dying, for example, has radical implications for the duty of the physician to be honest in disclosing a terminal diagnosis and for administering analgesia at a level that permits the patient to remain lucid. The preparation for the last rites requires certain behaviors not only for patients but also for providers.

At the same time, Catholic moral theology as articulated by the Church and its teachers has some implications that are not always well known to those outside the tradition. For example, the doctrine of double effect permits the administration of narcotic analgesia at high doses if necessary to relieve levels of pain that could interfere with one's religious preparation for death. Even the risk of a lethal side effect is clearly toler-ated. In contrast to Talmudic teaching, Catholic patients have no rigorous duty to preserve life, at least until the final moments when intervention would be seen as interfering with the divine will. Their doctrine of extra-ordinary means, now often called proportionality, accepts decisions to forgo life support even though the result will hasten death, a position that can be traced back into the history of Catholic medical morality.[65] Some of the most distinguished Catholic theologians have claimed that avant-garde, liberal definitions of death such as the higher-brain definition (which goes well beyond the now widely accepted whole-brain defini-tion) are acceptable.[66]

What is critical is that the physician schooled at the most advanced levels in Hippocratic and more recent professionally generated medical ethics but without serious training in Catholic moral theology should have no clue to understanding the teleological natural law as interpreted by the tradition of Catholic moral theology. Insofar as the natural law is believed to be knowable by reason, presumably the non-Catholic physi-cian should have access to some knowledge of the moral law but surely could not claim any expertise in interpreting its implications for the prac-tice of medicine. Moreover, the Catholic layperson, the patient in the doctor–patient relation, has at least as much claim to expertise in such interpretation.

Catholic natural law theory, while knowable by reason by any consci-entious person, is known only imperfectly through that method. Knowl-edge is believed to be supplemented by revelation through scripture, Church tradition, and the teachers of the Church. While the pope does not speak infallibly on matters of medical morality, he does speak author-itatively and commands serious attention by anyone claiming to stand in that tradition (and anyone else for that matter). Hence, since reason is supplemented by these revelatory sources, Catholic physicians and Catholic laypeople may believe they have advantage in understanding the moral law for medicine. A knowledgeable Catholic patient who is a serious student of the tradition may thus plausibly claim greater expertise on the natural moral law's implications for medical decision making than a member of the profession who lacks similar access to the tradition.

Certainly, for a Catholic who accepts the natural law doctrine and the associated roles for reason and revelation, medical professional groups can claim no special expertise in knowing the moral norms for the practice of medicine. Professional groups standing outside the Catholic tradition—including groups claiming to be grounded in the Hippocratic Oath—would be particularly poorly qualified to understand the proper basis for medical decision making in a Catholic context. It makes no sense for a serious Catholic patient to yield to the moral judgments of a physician. If that physician happens to be herself standing in the Catholic tradition, she is normally still theologically a layperson, one who would have to turn outside the medical profession to the authoritative interpreters of the tradition who would normally not be medical professionals.[67] It would be particularly irrational for a patient who claims to stand committed to Catholic moral theology and natural moral law theory to yield to a non-Catholic physician on matters of medical ethics or to subject himself to professionally generated codes of ethics that are articulated by persons or groups not purporting to have knowledge of the relevant moral church tradition—persons who, in fact, claim other metaethical commitments that point them to professional sources of knowledge rather than theological ones.

Philipp Melancthon

While Roman Catholic moral theology is the most consistent exemplar of a naturalist metaethics that relies on reason, at least in part, for knowledge of moral norms, some Protestant traditions also accept some versions of natural law thinking or otherwise give a place to the role of reason or other natural means of knowing the moral norms, including the norms that should govern medical decision making. To be sure, some branches of Protestantism are skeptical of the role of reason and other natural sources of knowledge available, in principle, to all people. By contrast, in spite of Barth and many Lutheran interpreters, some Protestants are more open to natural law approaches to ethics in which knowledge of moral norms is to some extent available to all through the use of reason. Luther's colleague at Wittenberg, Philipp Melancthon, recognized some capacity for humans to know the natural law by the use of reason. He saw the Ten Commandments as a summary of the natural law. His view, however, required that humans first accept by faith the first three commandments before the remainder could be the basis of an ethic knowable by reason.[68] That would seem to imply that, for a medical ethic that might be based on such an ethic, only those within the faith community would have the capacity to know what is morally required of health professionals and patients. If a modern Melancthon wanted to receive health care from providers who would base their ethical judgments on this natural law, he would have to rely on providers who were members of the community of faith or who relied on those within that community to establish the ethical norms. Nevertheless, in contrast to Luther, Melancthon has been described as reflecting "a more rational side of Protestantism."[69] He included into his ethical epistemology the notion that humans have had incorporated within them a "natural light," giving rise to certain "innate ideas" that can form the basis of moral judgments. Though darkened by the fall, the content of the natural moral law is given once again in the Ten Commandments.[70] In the following chapter I explore the implications of these "innate ideas" believed to be embedded in the human consciousness for a "common morality" that might serve as the basis of a secular medical ethic.

John Calvin

The reformed tradition provides a somewhat clearer example of the acceptance of the potential for natural law as a basis for a professional morality for health providers and patients (as well as for all other professions). Although some modern scholars have attempted to downplay Calvin's natural law, even pressing him in the direction of Barth, others insist he maintains a more robust commitment to the doctrine that divine law is available to humans for social and political purposes (including presumably medical ethical decision making).[71] At least in the civil kingdom, which presumably would include the realm of mainstream secular medicine as practiced in government-sponsored and -controlled hospitals, there is room for natural knowledge of the moral law that is to govern medical decision making and interactions between health professionals and patients across religious and secular communities. Thus, at least in some modern understandings of Calvinist theory, some Protestant as well as Catholic medical morality has a natural foundation that can be shared by the religiously committed and the secular world alike.

John Wesley

A final example of Protestant traditions open to some element of natural knowledge of the fundamentals of morality as it might govern professional practices including the practice of medicine can be found in John Wesley's Methodism. Methodism is known for a developed theory of knowledge known as the "quadrilateral."[72] It holds that theological knowledge (including knowledge of the basic principles of moral theology) can be known in four ways: scripture, tradition, reason, and experience.[73] Like most other Protestant denominations, Methodists have placed first emphasis on scriptural sources, but the quadrilateral incorporates sources of knowing the moral law that are remarkably similar to Roman Catholic doctrine. The addition that is unique is the creation of a place for experience. Wesley was heavily influenced by British empiricist philosophy.

Hence, Methodism, like most other mainstream Protestant denominations, can form an uneasy alliance with secular moral theories, especially those that rely on reason and experience even if it superimposes a requirement that divine grace is necessary for the functioning of the human will in the articulation of a set of moral norms that structure the assessment of human interactions and, in turn, provide a foundation for the more specialized subset of morality that governs the interactions of laypeople and professionals.

What is unacceptable is a theory of professional ethics that detaches the norms of professional conduct from the more fundamental overarching moral structure of all human conduct. Only after a more general moral theory is formulated so that the basic norms of conduct for evaluating the entire range of human actions is established can the members of society begin the more narrow project of deriving from those basic norms of conduct a more focused codification of the norms for lay–professional interactions.[74] Professional ethics cannot be conceptualized as a morality internal to a profession. Such an internal morality would not only cast out one-half—a critical half—of the lay–professional relation, it would also divorce the norms of professional conduct and the conduct of laypersons interacting with professionals from the more fundamental moral practices that govern all human behavior.

Thus, professional ethics is always an external morality. For the more fundamentalist and charismatic religious traditions, that external source is revelation. The norms of professional conduct are for revealed religion fundamentally incomprehensible to professional groups except as those norms are revealed, normally through the religious operatives and their special, privileged channels for acquiring knowledge of the divine law or will. For the religious traditions that incorporate natural means of knowing the moral law—reason or experience, for instance—the external source is more accessible to secular processes even if that knowledge is necessarily fallible and in need of summarizing guidance through scripture or other revelation.

What is critical is that the religious theories of moral epistemology that incorporate natural means of knowing provide an opening to dialogue and cooperation with secular sources that is fundamentally closed to the more sectarian religious traditions for which knowledge is, in principle, nonnatural—indeed, supernatural. For an alternative to Hippocratic and other professionally generated or articulated ethics for the professional–lay relation, we must turn to the possibility of a coalition between mainstream theological ethics with its natural epistemology and secular philosophical ethics.

SECULAR ETHICS AND PROFESSIONAL ETHICS

I N THE PREVIOUS CHAPTER we saw that religious moral epistemologies come in two forms: revealed and naturally knowable religious ethics. Those professionals and patients who accept one or another form of revealed religion should find themselves with a set of commitments that they believe should provide the bedrock of morality for their choices. Other traditions that have religious grounding claim that their knowledge of moral norms is available through natural processes of reason, experience, and common reflection on a moral tradition. Those religiously grounded metaethics should leave laypeople and professionals willing to enter into a common discourse with secular members of the moral community in a common quest for a set of moral norms to govern professional relations with laypeople.

Many laypeople and members of health professions, of course, do not claim to be religious. Religiously articulated ethics, whether revealed or natural, has no appeal to them. Religion has no claim on their loyalty when it comes to the foundation of ethics for professional practice. These people, however, will likely see themselves as standing in some secular tradition, or at least they will act as if they are members, whether they are aware of it or not. They will accept liberal political philosophy, libertarianism, communitarianism, or socialism in one of its varieties (democratic, totalitarian, or nationalistic).

The problem for these professionals is analogous to that of those who claim to stand in one of the religious groups. Each of these philosophical schools claims to have a theory about how ethics is generated or at least a normative theory about the norms of right action. For example, mainstream American physicians, nurses, pharmacists, and social workers are likely to acknowledge that they hold certain truths to be self-evident and that, among these, they accept that all people are created equal and endowed with certain inalienable rights. That core set of beliefs is the American version of liberal political philosophy accepted by our so-called Founding Fathers. Most health professionals licensed to practice their professions by various American government agencies tend to accept this American version of liberal political philosophy. Others may come down more strongly on the sole primacy of a principle of utility. They are utilitarian health professionals. Still others may commit to the primacy of the principle of autonomy. They are libertarian health professionals. Others with adequate training may admit to being Rawlsians, communitarians, or even Marxists. The problem for these secular physicians, like their religious brothers and sisters, is that these moral theories have metaethical and normative commitments that have nothing to do with Hippocratic and other professionally generated ethics. Rather than claiming that the morality for the practice of medicine must be "internal" to the practice derived by some pure reflection on the bare meaning of medicine or health, the plausible foundation for a morality for professional practice is necessarily "external" to the practice. It comes from the basic moral understanding articulated by various religious and secular worldviews.

When more basic questions about morality are addressed and answered about the ends of life and the duties humans have in social interactions with fellow humans, only then can we turn to the more narrow questions about how those who adopt a particular worldview understand how particular social roles like physician or patient should be governed.

Let's explore this conflict at the metaethical level, where the parallels between natural theology and the conflicts with Hippocratic and other professional moral theories will be apparent. (The conflicts at the normative level are equally dramatic.) Two major traditions in secular ethics have offered answers to the question of how we may know what is morally required: approaches based on reason and approaches based on experience or moral sense. Recently, efforts have been made to undercut the possible tension between these two approaches in what has sometimes been referred to as a "Common Morality" theory.

The Role of Reason

Many secular moral philosophers have relied on reason to establish the moral norms for a system of ethics. The eighteenth-century Enlightenment was a major contributor to the use of reason. One of the giant forces in the use of reason during this period was the German philosopher Immanuel Kant.

Immanuel Kant

Kant's method for establishing the norms of ethics relied on one of the strategies used by Catholics and certain Protestants—reason. As most college students know, Kant believed he could establish a set of moral maxims through the use of reason. Seeking maxims that one could act upon while simultaneously willing that they be universal laws governing human action, Kant believed he could identify certain behaviors that reason would require should be judged unethical.

One of the most serious moral problems of Hippocratic ethics is that it lacks any condemnation of lying to patients. In fact, historically it has often been claimed that physicians had a moral duty to lie to patients when speaking truthfully to them would do them harm. Hence, lying to patients was the professional norm when cancer was diagnosed and disclosure was judged by the physician to produce significant distress to the patient.[1]

Kant's maxim would judge such lying unethical regardless of the sup-posed distress to the patient.[2] Other critics of Hippocratic paternalism, such as Joseph Fletcher, the sometime Episcopal Christian medical eth-icist, would attack this Hippocratic paternalism on the grounds that it would produce bad consequences in the end.[3] One way or another, almost all nonprofessional commentators on the question of paternalistic lying to patients disagree with the Hippocratic answer. Such paternalistic lying by physicians has even been rejected by some later professional ethical codes, including the current American Medical Association code, which, since 1980, has committed the physician to dealing honestly with patients and colleagues without any patient-benefiting exception.[4]

What is critical for our purposes is not the overwhelming rejection of Hippocratic paternalism on the subject of truth-telling to patients. Rather, the critical difference is Kant's belief that the choice of a maxim is knowable by all through reason. While the Hippocratic and other pro-fessionally generated ethics start with the premise that the duty for physi-cians is determined or articulated by the professional group, those who claim ethics is a matter of reason claim that the maxims governing human conduct, including physician conduct, are knowable by all people capable of reason.

It is not that reason must dictate the same general maxim for all peo-ple in all roles. It may be that a nuanced ethic of truth-telling might identify certain circumstances and certain roles for which lying could be reasonable. To take an easy case, professional magicians are granted permission to lie to their audience when making deceptive claims about their tricks. To take a somewhat more complicated and serious example, perhaps it is reasonable that professionals working in clandestine intelli-gence for their governments are seen as having permission to lie or deceive. Similarly, parents may be given leeway to lie or deceive their small children in certain cases (although this example is particularly controversial).

What is important is not whether reason would permit violating the truth-telling maxim in any of these cases. What is important is that those who claim that moral maxims are knowable by reason commit to the proposition that the ethics of lying, including lying to patients, is accessible to all reasonable people, not merely to members of a particular professional group who have sole custody over the ethical norms for the members of their group. Unless defenders of professionally generated ethics can sustain the claim that only members of the profession have the ability to reason about the norms governing their behaviors, they cannot sustain the claim that the profession has sole custody of the ethics governing patient–physician relations.

John Rawls

In the twentieth century, at least in the United States, the philosopher most closely associated with the use of reason as a source of moral norms is John Rawls. His hypothetical social contract method is based on the premise that, using reason, one can imagine people coming together to form a social contract in which they ask what basic moral principles would be rational to accept if the contractors did not know their own unique and idiosyncratic positions. These principles would provide the basis for social institutions.[5]

Rawls is clear that his reason-based method is not meant to provide a decision tool for specific evaluations of individual actions—bedside choices for physicians, for example. However, the method is supposed to provide the principles governing basic social practices. Rawls is not as clear as he could be about what these basic social practices are. He eschews applying his principles to health care, for example. Nevertheless, many of his students have pressed the implications for social practices such as health care.[6] All of this work, purportedly teasing out the implications of reason for health care, offers norms that place heavy emphasis on the just distribution of health care and the duty of physicians to practice medicine within a context that somehow structures medicine to give people access to opportunities for their fair share of health care.

All these theorists produce moral frameworks for health care (including norms for physician behavior) that depart radically from the received traditional norms generated by the profession. As we have seen, the Hippocratic Oath is utterly silent on questions of access to health care. The Hippocratic core principle that the physician is to benefit the patient and protect the patient from harm implies the duty of the clinician to focus exclusively on the welfare of the patient and correlatively to exclude considerations that deal with the welfare of others in society.

Since the days of Thomas Percival, physicians have realized the serious deficiency of Hippocratic ethics in this regard. Percival, dealing with the dilemma of an epidemic at the Manchester Infirmary, saw fit to address matters of social ethics as well as obligations to individual patients. Following the best thinking of philosophers of the Scottish Enlightenment, he tended to offer social ethical perspectives that dealt exclusively with consequences. Even if he qualified his consequentialism, he did not offer a specific, detailed theory of the just distribution of health care the way followers of Rawls have attempted.

Once again, the point is not that social philosophers who rely on reason have offered the correct norms for physician conduct that can claim superiority over Hippocratic and other professionally generated norms. It seems clear that these more recent products of rationalist philosophers of medicine are superior to the alternative of ignoring social ethics for medicine. The critical issue is that, as with Kant, the use of reason as the method of knowing what is morally required is the authority for establishing norms. Reason provides the norms for professional and lay behavior, and that reasoning is not limited exclusively to members of the medical profession. Any reasonable person has standing to enter the conversation about the correct norms for social allocation of resources.

Limiting the conversation to members of the profession seems clearly to produce biased answers that come from limited perspective and exclusion of inputs from the overwhelming majority of reasonable people who are not members of the profession. I know of no reasonable person outside the medical profession (and precious few within it) who would be content in claiming that the ethics for medicine should remain silent on the just allocation of scarce medical resources. Any reasonable ethic for medicine must say something about how scarce resources should be allocated and about what the duty of the health professional is in the context of a just health care policy. Basing medical ethics on reason requires permitting all reasonable members of the moral community—lay and professional—to have a voice in forming that policy.

Experience and Sense Theories

The other major theory of the source of ethics, and therefore ethics for medical professionals, focuses on the senses. Empiricist metaethical presumptions run deep in accounts of the grounding of morality. Just as some religious ethics, such as Wesley's, include experience as a way of knowing moral norms, so secular theorists, sometimes touched by their underlying religious beliefs, hold to some model of sensory inputs.

The Scottish Enlightenment

The Scottish Enlightenment is an early highpoint. Francis Hutcheson was an early proponent of "moral sense theory."[7] A generation later Adam Smith expressed it in terms of "moral sentiments."[8] Infatuated by the discovery of the capacity of the human body to perceive through the physical senses, proponents posited, sometimes literally, sense receptors that permit the human to perceive the feelings of others, producing sympathy.

This led the Enlightenment figures to develop normative moral theories that emphasized the moral weight of benefits and harms experienced by other humans as like one's own. This became the foundation for modern social consequentialism.

The analogy with the Hippocratic ethic is dramatic. Hippocratism, at least in its modern form, views medical ethics as a moral relation between two people—health provider and patient. It is as if in all the world there are only two people interacting. The duty of the physician is to grasp the suffering of the patient and make choices that would benefit him. To be sure, the Hippocratic theory was dramatically one-sided; the physician was the one doing the perceiving of the other. The patient was passive. There is nothing in Hippocratic ethics about the patient as active perceiver of the physician. The patient's moral job was to follow doctor's orders.

The literature on compliance is directly derived from the Hippocratic notion of patient benefit. It rests on a confidence that somehow the physician is the best person to determine what is in the patient's interest (as the Oath says, "according to the physician's ability and judgment"). No matter that reasonable patients will gain a large part of their well-being by benefits in other areas of their lives. No matter that reasonable patients will evaluate the effects of medical interventions uniquely, and often differently than their physicians do. The Hippocratic physician is expected to focus on the patient before her and choose the regimen believed by the physician to be beneficial. It is critical at this point that Hippocratic clinicians see the impact of medical choices on others as out of bounds. This makes public health a difficult, counterintuitive concern for physicians. It makes human subjects research very implausible, requiring a complicated and controversial theory of "equipoise" to make the clinician's participation in human subjects' research morally palatable.[9] It makes physicians militantly loyal to their patients who contemplate gaming the resource allocation decisions of health insurance companies. (More than two-thirds of physicians reported that they would lie about a patient's diagnosis in order to gain insurance company payment for some treatment that they thought their patient could use.[10]) Transplant surgeons, knowing that their patients desperately need liver transplants, have been tempted to manipulate patient medical information in order to get them listed higher.

The ethical theorists of the Enlightenment recognized, often through their embracing of empathy for others, the moral imperative to factor the interests of third parties into medical decisions. Ideally that would happen without the aggregate social interests of others swamping the interests of the patient, a problem that utilitarian ethics grounded in the Enlightenment has difficulty handling, but somehow these third-party interests have to get on the agenda, something that the Hippocratic ethics of the medical profession has been reluctant to embrace.

When medical ethics was born in Edinburgh in about 1770, its most enlightened practitioner, physician/philosopher John Gregory, did not buy into the metaethical and normative theories of the medical profession.[11] He was remarkably disinterested in Hippocratic ethics. Hippocratic aphorisms were the focus of tests of medical students who were still required to demonstrate their ability to translate short bits of classical Greek, but one searches long and hard to find any reference in Gregory to the Hippocratic ethical tradition. He was an integral part of the Scottish Enlightenment's development of ethical theory. He reflects that social consequentialism in his medical ethics.

Ralph Barton Perry

The theory of moral knowledge pioneered by the figures of the Enlightenment is further developed in the twentieth century. Ethical naturalism is a twentieth-century view of the grounding of morality in analyzable natural properties. Gifford lecturer Ralph Barton Perry provides a good example of a more empirical form of naturalism. Perry was influenced by and was the biographer of earlier Gifford lecturer William James.[12] Both were professors at Harvard (James from 1873 to 1907 and Perry from 1902 to 1946—immediately after which he became the Gifford lecturer at Glasgow). Perry was also responsible for the posthumous collection of James's essays.[13]

Perry's Gifford lectures, published as *Realms of Value: A Critique of Human Civilization*, set out his moral theory including his understanding of morality as capable of being analyzed as a harmony of interests. Says Perry, "Morality is man's endeavor to harmonize conflicting interests."[14] He puts forward an understanding of morality that is naturalist; it defines morality as analyzable in empirically verifiable properties.[15]

My interest is not in Perry's specific formulation pertaining to the harmonious happiness of the group as the end of morality. That seems implausible. What is important is positioning Perry in the long line of proponents of empiricist naturalistic ethics. He understands knowledge of morality as empirical, as knowable through observation. Morality is "empirical in the full sense" if it is "a system of concepts verified by the data of human life."[16]

Roderick Firth

In 1952 Harvard philosopher Roderick Firth offered an empirical model for understanding the grounding of moral claims that continued the Enlightenment empiricist tradition and the empiricist commitments of Perry.[17] Firth understands moral knowledge in terms of perception and sets out to articulate the conditions under which perception of moral requiredness can be maximally accurate. He claims that a proposition is morally right to the extent that it would be perceived as correct by an ideal observer.

The ideal observer would have six key characteristics. He would have all the relevant, nonethical facts (be "omniscient"); be capable of visualizing the facts and all the consequences of possible acts (be "omnipercipient"); be disinterested, dispassionate, and consistent; and be normal in all other respects. To the extent that one possesses these characteristics, says Firth, one is capable of observing the moral reality and having knowledge of the moral norms. Of course, no ideal observer exists in reality. The beauty of the theory, however, is that it gives us a ready-made checklist for the characteristics we should strive for in order to perceive ethical requiredness correctly.

The shocking implication is that the individual physician or even committees of professional organizations fail miserably to approach the ideals reflected in these criteria. The individual physician is lacking major categories of information needed by the ideal observer. First, they generally have little or no information about the major nonmedical interests of patients. Any patient deciding what treatment would be most beneficial would give prominent place in the calculation of her interests to the psychological, economic, social, familial, legal, aesthetic, and religious agenda. Normally, the physician at the bedside is dreadfully lacking in knowledge about these nonmedical interests of the patient.

Even within the medical sphere, different medical goals will require different medical treatment choices. Medical goals are pluralistic. They can involve prevention of death, cure of disease, relief of suffering, and preservation and promotion of health. In many cases the choice of the correct medical treatment will depend on the relative priority given these diverse and often conflicting goals. There is no reason to assume that the physician's balancing of these competing claims is the definitively correct one. Different patients with different priorities within the medical sphere will correctly perceive different treatments as serving their best interest. When the patient's nonmedical values are factored in, it is pure hubris for a physician to suggest he could possibly know what is best for the patient. Even asking the patient to explain her values will at best give the physician at the bedside only a rudimentary, distorted look at what the patient believes will make her life go best. The physician is far from the ideal observer that Firth would seek to determine what is morally required.

Shifting to a collectivity of physicians such as we find in the typical committee that takes on the task of writing a code of ethics for a profession does not really solve the problem. It might eliminate the personal, idiosyncratic biases of the individual provider but does nothing whatsoever to correct the systematic biases that a committee of physicians would bring to the table. For example, one issue any committee of code writers would have to address is how to balance medical and nonmedical welfare. It would be absurd to claim that a committee made up entirely of physicians (which is the normal makeup of the professional association code writers) could possibly be unbiased in deciding how to balance medical and nonmedical interests.

Similar problems arise at the level of constructing a system of normative ethical principles. Physicians have historically gravitated toward the normative theories of consequentialism. In spite of the weighty presence of deontological theories, at least since the days of Kant and democratic liberal political theories of human rights, only in the past few years have deontological concerns and rights theories put in any appearance in any professional medical ethical code. It is not until 1980 that the first occurrence of the word "rights" appears in any professionally generated medical ethical code. Any committee made up entirely of physicians has to provide a very biased sample in the choice of a normative ethical theory.

Omnipercipience is not a characteristic of professional code writers either. Their visualization of outcomes of actions is distorted by the dominance of the biomedical sphere in their worldview. It is sometimes argued that physician code writers have the advantage of long experience as physicians. They have witnessed the plight of patients suffering many maladies. It is even suggested that patients and other medical laypeople lack this experience. The problem, however, is that long experience as a medical professional may actually distort one's vision. The worldview of health professionals is overmedicalized. Many people they encounter are sick and suffering. In some cases, patients are perceived as out of control and mentally impaired by their illness (even if most patients today are either perfectly healthy—seeing a doctor for an annual check-up, an employment interview, or immunizations—but not at all sick or impaired).[18]

Physicians are trained to be disinterested and dispassionate, but they are also encouraged to be concerned and compassionate. They are trained for detached concern, to use Renée C. Fox's term.[19] While state-licensed physicians may at first appear "normal" in all other relevant respects, they are upon reflection actually an atypical lot. They are successful academically, consistent overachievers, more oriented to the sciences, and—at least until recently—overwhelmingly Caucasian, upper-middle class, older than mid-age males. A collection of these atypical characters gathered together to write a code of ethics is not collectively much like Firth's ideal observer. It is an atypical, distorted sample of a specialized section of the public. They may once have thought like patients, but that naivete has long since been forced out of them.

The empirical theories of moral sense and the ideal observer are simply incompatible with giving the individual physician or the professional association committee of physicians the role of exclusive authorities in knowing what is moral in the doctor–patient relation. A case might be made that the physician is the expert on the medical facts related to a patient's condition. Even that claim poses some problems for those who in the postmodern world reject the claim that facts, such as medical facts, can be known in a value-free way.[20] If physicians bring special sets of values to their description of the medical facts, and if fact descriptions are always inevitably dependent on the speaker's system of beliefs and values, then there is reason to be concerned if a physician or group of physicians claims unbiased expertise in describing the medical facts.

Even if we assume that the physician is the presumed expert in describing the medical facts, the presumption that the individual physician or a group of physicians has expertise in developing a moral code for their profession is baseless. To the contrary, we have every reason to believe that physicians (or any other specialized group) would be expected to make distorted choices when they put forward a moral code. In the case of classical professional medical ethics, their theory is unacceptably overcommitted to consequences at the expense of nonconsequentialistic moral principles such as autonomy and justice. Their theory is unacceptably overcommitted to the consequences for the patient to the exclusion of those for all others in society. Their theory is unacceptably overcommitted to the place of the physician in deciding what counts as a good consequence for the patient. There is nothing in ideal observer theory that would support using a committee made up entirely of members of a single profession to pick the proper principles for the patient–physician relation.

Common Morality

I am by no means suggesting that the secular philosophical theories offer a common view about moral epistemology. Theories that emphasize reason have important differences from those that emphasize experience and moral sense. What is obvious, however, is that neither reason-based nor empirically based theories could possibly support professionally generated or articulated ethics for a profession. Professional ethics must come later in the process of the development of a moral code. The process has to involve several stages.

First, using reason and experience, perhaps aided by religious notions of revelation, we must have agreement on a general ethical system with a short set of norms (principles or rules or rights) that should provide the basis for moral evaluation of all human actions. Then, after all members of the moral community have available to them a moral system, a normative ethic that provides a basis for the general practices underlying all human conduct, they can set out to develop more specialized ethics for the members of varying professional groups and their clients. The members of the society, laypeople and professionals, will have to specify the implications of the more basic ethical system for professional conduct. Presumably, an ethical specification or code of conduct should be developed for each profession. The development of these specialized ethics for lay and professional conduct when these parties interact will not be merely a "professional" ethic. It will be an ethic for both laypeople and professionals, and both groups should have a voice in agreeing on the norms for these parties when they interact. The moral conduct of professionals must be evaluated by standards that are equally accessible to laypeople. Those laypeople have a legitimate role in articulating what those norms are.

It seems reasonable that a society would provide a general set of ethical norms for professional and lay conduct for each profession that would apply to all participants in any professional service. In addition, however, more specialized "sectarian" groups may choose to impose further moral obligations. In more sectarian health care systems—those of the Christian Scientists, Jehovah's Witnesses, Seventh Day Adventists, and City of Faith Medical Center—the medical laypeople (including the medical laypeople who are the theologians of these traditions) will work with members of the profession who stand within these groups to articulate the goals of medicine as well as the ways their professional practitioners can advance those goals.

In more secular medicine, the norms will be articulated by the medical laypeople working with members of the profession. They will all draw on their religious and secular views about natural sources of moral knowledge to develop a general moral system for all human conduct, and will then extract from that general set of norms some more specialized norms for various professionals and laypeople who must interact in specific subspheres.

What makes no sense, what is irrational, is a system in which members of a single profession all come together to select and impose a set of moral norms on the laypeople obtaining services from that profession, regardless of the moral commitments of various professionals to religious and secular ethical systems. Individual members of any profession will be simultaneously members of the various religious and secular systems of belief from which they might derive their judgments about the proper set of moral principles. There is no reason to believe that the members of the profession who bring with them diverse religious and philosophical beliefs should agree on the norms for the profession except insofar as their underlying groups can also agree.

We can imagine a meeting of the profession—for example, a meeting in Geneva of the representatives of the World Medical Association—in which Catholic, feminist, Marxist, Buddhist, Orthodox Jewish, and secular liberal physicians come together to try to agree on a single, all-purpose set of norms for the practice of medicine. The result should be an ethical Babel, a chaos of conflicting moral points of view producing only the most banal platitudes. There is no reason why these participants should agree on the moral duties of physicians or patients unless they start with a preexisting set of agreed-upon norms for the more general conduct of human existence. Moreover, there is not necessarily any need for there to be any common agreement.

If the members of the profession fail to replicate the characteristics of ideal observers, they should not be expected to gravitate toward a single correct set of moral norms. The key for a general ethic for a health profession (or any profession) is whether an underlying ground for a moral code can be perceived or discovered by reason, common human experience, or some other general moral epistemology. The most recent developments in medical ethics that suggest such a ground come from the theory of the "common morality." Two teams of scholars have been giving serious attention to this notion for the past decade, one group associated with Dartmouth College and another team associated with Georgetown University's Kennedy Institute of Ethics.

The Dartmouth Group: Gert, Culver, and Clouser

A team of scholars, all of whom have had some association with Dartmouth College, has put forward in several places a notion of a common morality.[21] Their core claim is that there is widespread—indeed, universal—agreement on most moral matters. As they claim, "Everyone agrees that such actions as killing, causing pain or disability, and depriving of freedom or pleasure are immoral unless one has an adequate justification for doing them."[22] They add that everyone also agrees that "deceiving, breaking a promise, cheating, breaking the law, and neglecting one's duties also need justification in order not to be immoral."[23] They note that people do disagree about the scope of morality—whether the killing prohibition, for instance, applies to fetuses and nonhuman animals or merely to postnatal humans. They also acknowledge that justifications can be put forward to override these moral prohibitions and, further, that people disagree about what counts as an adequate moral justification. Nevertheless, they claim that disagreements about what counts as a justification for an exception do not cloud the agreement that some justification is needed for these actions.

Similarly, they claim that all agree that "what counts as an adequate justification for one person must be an adequate justification for anyone else in the same situation."[24] Thus, they claim that everyone accepts the notion that ethical propositions must be impartial. They also claim that, contrary to some professionally generated ethics, an ethical system must be public. All persons to whom it applies must understand it. Moreover (and here they introduce a rationality criterion), it must not be irrational for any persons to accept being guided and judged by such a system. Thus, they conclude, morality must be a public system that applies to all moral agents. "All people are subject to morality simply by virtue of being rational persons who are responsible for their actions."[25]

The Kennedy Institute Group

A somewhat similar idea using the same term has emerged among scholars associated with the Kennedy Institute of Ethics at Georgetown University.[26] Tom Beauchamp and James Childress introduce the concept in the 1994 fourth edition of *The Principles of Biomedical Ethics* and expand the coverage greatly in the fifth edition (2001). They hold that "all morally serious persons" share a set of norms. They call this set of norms the "common morality."[27] They note that this shared set of norms can be expressed variously in the language of human rights, moral obligations, or moral virtues. This universal common morality stands in contrast with community-specific morality, the morality of specific cultural, religious, and institutional sources, including, perhaps, the morality of particular professional organizations.

Beauchamp and Childress distinguish between normative and empirical claims related to the common morality. Normatively, the claim is that the common morality establishes obligatory standards for everyone. If a norm, no matter how specific or concrete, is part of the common morality, it is universal in the sense that it applies to everyone. The issue here is not whether the norm is situational, that is, fine-tuned so that different rules apply in different situations. Rather, the claim is that a judgment, no matter how situational, should be seen by all as morally binding. Thus, a rule about getting informed consent may vary depending on the circumstances of persons, places, times, and culture. It may take into account the mental capability of the patient, the time constraints of an emergency, or whether patient and provider share a common language, but a claim that a consent with certain characteristics is or is not morally required in a specific circumstance is a claim that should be evaluated the same by all people; that is, they should evaluate it the same if they had perfect capacities to reason about the issues or were ideal moral observers of the situation. Two people observing the same consent process who disagree about whether it was morally acceptable have a real disagreement. Both would agree that at least one of them must be wrong. By contrast, two people who disagree about whether a food tastes good

may both be expressing legitimate opinions that can be held simultaneously without contradiction. They would each merely be expressing their
opinion about food taste, whereas disagreements about the morality of a
medical action such as getting consent suggest a conflict that begs for
resolution.

Sometimes the common morality thesis is also taken to be an empirical claim—that all persons (or all serious persons) actually do agree on
some basic set of moral norms. This empirical claim is controversial and
hard to establish. It is the basis of many of the criticisms of common
morality theory.[28] Surely, it is obviously false to claim that all humans in
fact share a belief in a common set of moral norms. Some humans lack
the capacity to hold any moral norms. Others, while having such a capacity, have never cultivated a set of norms and can be said to live amoral
lives. They might be said to be moral infants lacking any set of norms.
Still others are selectively moral but lack anything like a full-blown set
of norms that could be associated with a common morality. Just as some
observers of the physical world are so untrained that they make simple
mistakes that are clearly incorrect, likewise some observers of the moral
world are similarly naive or biased. The claim is not that all persons share
a set of moral norms but that they would share such a set if they were
only minimally skilled at reason or observation.

This claim runs the risk of being circular, of suggesting that anyone
who does not affirm some common set of norms is unreasonable or is
not serious about morality. That surely is not an adequate foundation
for the claim that a common morality exists. Rather, the claim is based
simultaneously on empirical facts of morality and speculation about what
people would believe is adequately rational and serious.

The claim is analogous to the one scientists would make about the
earth being flat or about a law of gravity. Obviously, not everyone believes
the earth is a sphere or that, within certain limits, bodies attract one
another in an orderly way related to the masses and the distance between
them. The claim of a scientist is, rather, that the earth is roughly spheri-
cal and would not be understood to be flat by anyone who is adequately
serious in thinking about the question based on standard observations

that are beyond dispute. The claim is that someone who held that the earth is flat would be making a mistake and that the critic of the claim believes that the claimant could be convinced to adjust the claim if only he or she were serious in assessing the data.

Likewise, defenders of the common morality thesis claim that a set of moral norms exists that would be affirmed by anyone who was serious in assessing the data. One critical issue, however, is that the thesis is a claim about some "pretheoretical" insights that, as such, are unsystematized and not yet reduced to a theoretical system. This means that, although there is a common awareness of the norms, there is not necessarily agreement on how those norms can be described and organized into an ethical theory. Common morality theorists agree that moral theory is something that comes later. It is constructed by human theorists or cultural groups that must impose a language and a set of concepts to organize the pretheoretical insights.

Defenders of the common morality thesis generally acknowledge that theory construction is necessarily dependent on language, culture, and beliefs. An infinite number of theoretical constructs could be devised to account for our pretheoretical insights, and these theoretical constructs may not all sound exactly the same. Moreover, our pretheoretical insights, the raw data of a moral sense theory or the initial premises of a rationalist's theory, may conflict with one another, and no one claims that common morality includes agreement upon how the conflicts ought to be resolved.

Everyone seems to agree that the killing of humans (and perhaps certain other species) is morally problematic. How different theories describe the killing will be endlessly variable. Some will claim that all human life is precious in its every moment, so any shortening of life is morally problematic. Others may distinguish between killing and letting die, between murder and other forms of killing, between direct killing and indirect killing, and so forth.

Everyone also agrees that pain is a harm, and that it should be avoided. Some may describe pain as a burden, others as an evil. Some may distinguish between pain and suffering, or between pain and hurt. Some may construct theories in which only harm is to be avoided while others may claim that not only is harm to be avoided but good is also to be produced. There are endless accounts of how the avoiding of harm and the production of good relate to one another, and different theories will provide different constructions of that relation.

Because avoiding harms may shorten life in some situations, any moral theory will have to provide an account of what should happen when two pretheoretical moral insights appear to conflict. Is an exception created to the prohibition on killing when the killing is necessary to avoid the harm of pain, or does the prohibition survive the reasonable desire to avoid the harm of pain? The common morality thesis does not suggest that there will be agreement on the reasons why exceptions to some moral rules are justified. It does not claim that there is cross-theory consistency in moral terminology. What is claimed is that people who are reasonable or serious about morality would have available to them some common set of moral insights from which they could begin their theory construction and code writing. Also implied is the conviction that any general moral theory must somehow be in accord with these pretheoretical moral insights.

National Commission for the Protection of Human Subjects

One of the important examples in which common morality seems to have provided a foundation for producing a shared set of moral principles among a wide range of religious and secular theories arose in the National Commission for the Protection of Human Subjects of Biomedical and Behavioral Research, the eleven-member federal commission in the United States in the 1970s and 1980s that was mandated by federal law to produce an ethical framework for evaluating research involving human subjects.[29] The commission had the task of assessing such research in the light of exposés of ethically controversial research including the Tuskegee syphilis study, in which men diagnosed with syphilis were intentionally left untreated for a period of decades in order to study the effect of lack of treatment.[30] Although it was argued that there were no treatments recognized to be beneficial when the trial began in 1932, the trial continued until 1972, when treatments were clearly available that could have been used.

The controversy surrounding this trial and many others like it led to hearings before Sen. Ted Kennedy's Senate Health Subcommittee.[31] I was at the Hastings Center in New York at that time and was delegated to work with the subcommittee staff to plan hearings.[32] I ended up testifying at the hearings as well.[33] Those hearings gave rise to the legislation that mandated the commission and the first-ever federal requirement to produce a specific ethical framework for a government policy.

The result was the Belmont Report, which set out three principles—respect for persons, beneficence, and justice—as the foundation of policy to protect human subjects. Although these three principles may look different from other lists of principles, including the four principles of Beauchamp and Childress, I argue in the following that all of the normative ethical theories of the major contemporary bioethics theorists, including Beauchamp and Childress; Gert, Culver, and Clouser; the *Belmont Report*, and the Rice theorists; Baruch Brody and even Tristram Engelhardt; and the British contributors W. D. Ross and Ranaan Gillon as well as my own general medical ethical theory should be understood as theories reflecting the same underlying pretheoretical common morality.

The seemingly overwhelming task was to produce a single consensus document on ethical principles that would be usable in the nation that was famously proud of its pluralism. It had to satisfy physicians, researchers, and other health professionals as well as laypeople. It had to satisfy people of the full range of religious denominations as well as secular people.

The commission was rigorously pluralistic. By law, the majority had to be laypeople rather than health professionals. It included three physicians, including its chair, Kenneth Ryan. It included a former Jesuit priest with a PhD focusing in medical ethics. It included a Protestant laywoman trained in theological ethics focusing on medicine. It included a number of leaders with no conspicuous religious affiliation. Its staff and consultants included a wide range of academic disciplines, religious orientations, and philosophical commitments.

Had the commission been asked to agree on the foundational source of ethical norms, chaos would have resulted. Religious claims grounding ethics in the will, judgment, or natural law of the deity would have conflicted with Kantian and Humean accounts. The commission attempted no statement on the foundation or source of ethical norms but instead agreed upon the three principles that could be accepted by all members regardless of religious or philosophical commitments. It was not irrelevant that Tom Beauchamp was among the commission staff developing the report. Common moral insights led to convergence around the three principles, even if some commissioners and staff would have used differing language or differing accounts of the moral content of and even the number of the principles. As a broad framework providing a basis for public moral discussion of human clinical trials, the Belmont Report's three principles have served us well for more than twenty-five years.[34] There is beginning to be hope for a morality of medicine stemming from religious ethics that have a natural epistemology grounded in reason and experience converging with secular ethics that affirm similar epistemological theories. In the final chapter of this volume I set out the claim that, in fact, religious and secular medical ethics, within the limits of human fallibility, are converging around a normative moral theory that reasonable laypeople and professionals can support as an alternative to professionally generated or professionally articulated ethics such as the Hippocratic Oath.

CHAPTER

7

FALLIBILISM AND THE CONVERGENCE HYPOTHESIS

I SEE NO HOPE for the Hippocratic ethic or similar professional ethics. The Hippocratic ethic is dead. Some alternative foundation for a medical ethic is needed. One option for those laypeople and professionals who accept religiously mediated sources of revelation—via scripture or direct mystical communication from the deity to some individual human—is for laypeople who believe they have a source of divine revelation of the moral law to get together with health professionals who share the same revelatory beliefs. That option, unfortunately, only works for those with sectarian beliefs who are willing to develop alternative, religiously based health care systems. The only problems that will arise will be the cases in which the revealed moral obligations conflict with the norms of the broader society.

A second option is available for the large portion of the lay and professional populations that do not have a divine moral system revealed to them and should not be content to accept the Hippocratic or other professionally produced system. In the spirit of the Gifford mandate, there may be natural sources available for grounding moral norms. The focus here is not on natural theology to demonstrate the existence and nature

159

of God by natural scientific means. Rather, our focus is on the use of natural means to know what religious people might claim is the divine moral law and what secular people might claim are moral norms knowable by reason or experience.

The Convergence Hypothesis

The common morality claim provides a context for proposing what can be called a "convergence hypothesis": that religious ethics knowable by natural means of reason and experience can produce normative moral theories that converge with secular ethical systems with natural epistemologies knowable by similar means. Even if religious ethics superimposes a metaethic involving a deity's will or creation or law and a secular ethic eschews any such theological trappings, it may be that the moral norms turn out to be, if not identical, at least similar enough that, in the spirit of the US National Commission, the two main categories of ethics can share the same or similar pretheoretical moral insights. Not only that, it may turn out that the theories that are constructed to systematize these pretheoretical insights overlap sufficiently and share enough in common that they provide common ground for a single normative framework. This framework would be publicly accessible, not the sole custody of a professional group that claims to be able to impose it on its own members, regardless of their competing loyalties to religious or philosophical traditions, as well as on the laypeople who are inevitably the clients of professionals and are necessarily the recipients of actions that result from the professional's moral choices.

Fallibilism

Before launching a final account of what this convergence might look like and why the major contemporary theories of normative action support the convergence hypothesis, however, one critical piece of the theory needs to be added. Modern philosophical epistemologies are comfortable with the doctrine of fallibilism, the notion that there is no certain knowledge. This is surely true in morality as well as science. Postmodern constructivists add to this more traditional uncertainty the idea that accounts of knowledge, even if from within a realist framework, require socially constructed linguistic conventions. Descriptions are so nuanced and complex that, even bracketing the fallibility that is inevitable, different people describing the same observed reality will identify different features of that reality as important. Only those features that are important enough will rise to the level that they are included in their accounts. This is surely true in describing our shared pretheoretical moral data as well as our accounts of physical reality. Thus, any descriptions of reality will be dependent upon the describer's beliefs and values. This is what William Stempsey and I have called "value-dependent realism."[1] These inevitable variations in accounts of the moral reality that depend on systems of belief and value are, of course, supplemented by the more traditional problems of the inevitable bias that comes from our limits as human observers.

These same problems arise in religious accounts of moral norms. Even if we assume there is a common morality that provides the data in a pretheoretical form, religious ethicists must construct their accounts of the moral norms. They must choose language and identify the important features of that reality to bring forward as significant.

Religious ethics in its natural form that relies on reason and experience, perhaps supplemented by revelation, faces an even more critical problem. Christian theology always incorporates some form of a doctrine of the fall of man, some notion that the human in his or her present condition inevitably is limited and fallible. This surely must apply to human accounts of the natural moral order as understood by the theological ethicists and as they apply those accounts to professional ethics for their tradition. The implication is that moral knowledge for the theological ethicist is at least as limited as it is for the philosopher who relies on natural epistemologies.

These constructivist notions of how a theory must be created from linguistic choices and under the guidance of what is considered important by a system of belief and value are more than enough to account for the variations in the normative theories that religious and secular ethicists put forward and for their implications for professional ethics. These inevitable variations attributable to the human construction of theory and the fallibility of human reason do more than explain the variations in bioethical normative theory; they also call out for substantial tolerance for differences in moral conclusions in the application of bioethical principles to specific problem solving. Especially when principles conflict so that the final duty proper has to be discerned from some theory of how to resolve conflict among principles, fallible humans are inevitably uncertain that their conclusions are correct and their opponent in moral debate is wrong. This problem is exacerbated by the dilemma of having to determine to whom moral duties are owed. As we have seen, common morality theory does not provide a mechanism for knowing who among us is a proper bearer of moral claims. Fetuses, embryos, the human in the ambiguous period near death, and nonhuman animals all pose problems for bioethical theory, not because we doubt what the norms are and not because we are uncertain how to resolve conflicts among the norms, but because we are uncertain to whom the norms apply. Even if we are certain that killing is a characteristic of actions that tends to make those actions wrong, we are uncertain whether the concept applies to embryos, fetuses, nonhuman animals, and humans with dead brains and beating hearts.

In summary, there are good grounds for hope that those brands of religious ethics that rely on natural means of knowledge of the moral norms can converge with those brands of secular ethics that rely on analogous means of knowledge of the moral norms, but human fallibility requires humility about the certainty that those norms are described properly. When that fallibility is combined with the inevitable variations in description that come from the human activity of theory construction, the need to develop strategies for resolving conflict among norms, and the need for determining to whom at the margins the norms are to apply, then humans—whether working in religious or secular worlds—must allow great room for error in their moral conclusions. Even though it is irrational for laypeople to be subjected to the privately generated and articulated norms of a professional group, and even though professionals themselves should turn outside the profession for the knowledge of the norms that should govern their practice, both laypeople and professionals must remain humble in the uncertainty that their version of the norms for lay–professional relations is the correct one.

This problem can be illustrated first in the cluster of normative ethical theories in bioethics that produce overlapping packages of norms while leaving clear differences in their theories. After considering this cluster of overlapping normative theories as an alternative to professionally gen-erated ethics for professional practice, I turn, finally, to the Universal Declaration of Human Rights and the related Universal Declaration on Bioethics and Human Rights as models for the proper negotiation of a convergence of religious and secular norms for the professional practice of medicine and the other health care professions.

Convergence Illustrated in Principle-Based and Similar Normative Theories

We have seen that both religious and secular normative ethics that rely on natural means of knowing—reason or experience—now have available a notion of common morality that supplies the "data" for theory construc-tion. These pretheoretical data points are known by asking what is ratio-nal or what is known by intuition or perception. In the end it may make little difference which set of metaphors is chosen. The claim is that one way or another, theorists constructing normative ethics have a small set of moral norms made available to them with which they can begin to build a theoretical account of the norms as they "perceive" them or find them irrational to resist.

Someone working in contemporary biomedical ethics cannot escape the awareness that several theories are available that rely on closely over-lapping and similar concepts. The fact that they are different in their detail may lead some to conclude that there is, in the end, no conver-gence, that each theorist comes up with his or her own package of norms independent of some unifying underlying moral reality. On the other hand, a closer look at these theories may reveal that, within the limits of human fallibility and variation in concept construction, these normative theories do, in fact, converge substantially. Let us start with the well-known four-principle version articulated by Beauchamp and Childress and adopted by Raanan Gillon, and compare it with theories by Mill, Engelhardt, the *Belmont Report*, Baruch Brody, W. D. Ross, my own theory, and that of Gert and his Dartmouth colleagues. (The results are summarized in table 7.1.)

Contemporary normative bioethics outside of professional ethics is represented by some single-principle theories (such as Mill's utilitarian principle or various libertarian views), the two-principle theory of Engelhardt, the three-principle theory of the *Belmont Report*, the classic four-principle theory of Beauchamp and Childress and of Gillon, the five "conflicting appeals" approach of Baruch Brody, the six prima facie duties of W. D. Ross, my own seven-principle theory, and finally the ten rules of Gert and his colleagues. This would seem to offer a strong case for chaos in normative bioethical theory rather than convergence explained by the claim that all are working from some common pretheoretical moral insights. A closer look, however, reveals a more complicated story.

Beauchamp–Childress and Gillon Compared with the *Belmont Report*: Four Principles or Three?

Let us start with the four principles of Beauchamp and Childress and the use of their principles by Gillon in the major text *The Principles of Health Care Ethics*.[2] These both put forward the now-famous four principles: beneficence, nonmaleficence, respect for autonomy, and justice. These could be compared with the three principles of the *Belmont Report*: respect for persons, beneficence, and justice.[3] Two differences are apparent, aside from the fact that one list contains four items and the other three. Respect for autonomy is replaced by "respect for persons" and nonmaleficence is omitted. These differences are of some importance, but that importance should not be overemphasized.

Table 7.1: Ethical Principles

Generic Name for Principle	Utilitarianism 1 Principle	Engelhardt 2 Principles	Belmont Report 3 Principles	Beauchamp & Childress 4 Principles	Brody 5 Conflicting Appeals	W. D. Ross 6 Prima Facie Duties	Veatch 7 Principles	Gert, Culver, Clouser 10 Rules
	1. Utility			Consequence-Maximizing Principles				
Beneficence	(Beneficence)	2. Beneficence	1. Beneficence	1. Beneficence	1. Consequence 5a. Cost-effectiveness	4. Beneficence 5. Self-improvement	1. Beneficence	
Nonmaleficence	(Nonmaleficence)			2. Nonmaleficence	2b. Not to have injury inflicted	6. Not injuring	2. Nonmaleficence	2. Don't cause pain 3. Do not disable 5. Do not deprive of pleasure
			Duty-Based (Deontological or Respect for Persons) Principles					
		2. Respect for persons			3. Respect for persons 2. Rights	Respect for persons principles		
Autonomy	(Respecting autonomy tends to maximize utility)	1. Permission	(Autonomy)	3. Respect for autonomy	2d. To decide 2e. To refuse health care		4. Autonomy	4. Do not deprive of freedom
Fidelity			(Promise-keeping)			1. Fidelity 1a. Promises	3. Fidelity	7. Keep promises 9. Obey the law 10. Do your duty
Veracity			(Veracity)			1a. Not lying	5. Veracity	6. Do not deceive 8. Do not cheat
Killing					2a. Not to be killed		6. Avoiding killing	1. Do not kill
Justice	(Just distribution tends to maximize utility)		3. Justice	4. Justice	5b. Justice	3. Justice	7. Justice	
Other principles					[4. Virtues]	1b. Gratitude 2. Reparation	[8. Gratitude] [9. Reparation]	

Respect for autonomy may sound like a synonym for "respect for persons," but the former, the Beauchamp–Childress term, implies that it is only a person's autonomy that is to be respected, which raises the question of whether other aspects of a person also should command respect and whether nonautonomous persons also command respect. Since one might still owe loyalty (faithfulness) or veracity to nonautonomous persons, the term "respect for autonomy" leaves open the ethics of certain other Kantian concerns that may not be captured adequately by the notion of autonomy.

The second difference is that the *Belmont Report* commits only to beneficence whereas Beauchamp and Childress include both principles of beneficence and nonmaleficence. The *Belmont Report* seems to cover for this by making clear that it considers both positive and negative aspects of beneficence. One can, so to speak, act in such a way that one produces negative beneficence, an awkward expression perhaps, but one that allows for considerations of harms or setbacks to people's interests.

What *Belmont's* formulation omits, however, is an easy vocabulary for addressing the moral relation between doing good and avoiding harm. The explicit use of the two terms makes that potentially important moral discussion much easier. For example, the nineteenth-century slogan "primum non nocere," which is often mistakenly taken to be Hippocratic, is most easily understood to have moral force if "first of all, do no harm" is understood as requiring a rank-ordering of nonmaleficence over beneficence so that one is first obligated to avoid doing harm before one takes up the question of whether one can do good. This is morally different from the Hippocratic form "benefit and do no harm" (without any indication of a "first of all" priority to nonmaleficence).

There are other issues of normative ethics that can be addressed much more easily if one has the two terms, beneficence and nonmaleficence, in one's moral vocabulary. Among consequence-oriented normative theories, there is more than one way of combining benefits and harms to determine one's moral duty. One can subtract the estimated harms from the estimated benefits, producing a net utility in Benthamite fashion, but one could also calculate the ratio of benefit to harm and strive to maximize the ratio. Many bedside clinicians think in ratio terms when they calculate treatment choices, especially when a high-risk/high-gain experimental treatment is compared with a low-risk/low-gain standard treatment. In such a comparison, if the benefit/harm ratios are seen as the same, a randomized clinical trial is considered justified. That condition, called "equipoise," is often considered a moral prerequisite for an ethically justified randomization.[4] The critical fact is that equalizing the benefit/harm ratios will, in these cases, not equalize net benefits calculated by subtracting expected harms from expected benefits. If both ratios are the same while both numerator and denominator are smaller in the case of the standard treatment, then the net utility will be smaller. In this case, a Benthamite would feel obliged to choose the experimental treatment while the ratio calculator would see the two options as tied. Having the terms "beneficence" and "nonmaleficence" makes it easier to discuss the morality of the relation between producing benefits and avoiding harms.

In spite of these marginal differences between the Beauchamp–Childress four principles and the *Belmont* three, it is easy to see that the two normative theories are providing accounts of the same or a similar moral reality. They simply provide slightly different linguistic conventions to describe the moral terrain. It is easier and more elegant to have the two terms—"beneficence" and "nonmaleficence"—available, but with more work and more words one could discuss the moral issues using the *Belmont* linguistic conventions. However, what about the other normative theories?

Utilitarianism, Libertarianism, and Hippocratic Theories: Single-Principle Theories

Utilitarianism Several normative theories solve the problem of conflict among moral principles by reducing all of ethics to a single principle. Utilitarianism is probably the most important of these. After collapsing beneficence and nonmaleficence into a single principle of utility maximizing, utilitarians claim that this principle is the only normative criterion in ethics. In the hands of a sophisticated utilitarian equipped with notions of rule utility, complex strategies for calculating qualitatively different utilities, and subtle estimates of the psychological effects of various policies, many, perhaps most, moral intuitions can be accounted for by utilitarians. Still, problems exist.

One problem is that some of the normal moral insights of the common morality have to be accounted for by converting them into utilitarian language. Both respect of autonomy and justice can be packed into utilitarian theory. Mill explains our inclination to want to favor the worst off by noting that decreasing marginal utility means that it is usually utility maximizing to provide benefits to the worst off.[5] (A cash gift to a poor person can easily do more good than the same-sized gift to a millionaire.)

In health care, however, this normal decreasing marginal utility from benefiting better-off persons sometimes does not work. Transplanting livers to healthier persons often does more good than targeting those with the worst liver disease. The worst off may be so sick that they will die even after receiving a new liver. The chronically ill with multiple illnesses may be the worst off and still very inefficient to treat. Utilitarians follow these facts to their conclusion that, in such cases, it is immoral to benefit the worst off. Typically, those who incorporate a principle of justice will feel some moral pull in the direction of helping the worst off even if it is not utility maximizing. Having a separate principle of justice in one's moral account of the common morality at least permits discussion of the relative importance of benefiting the worst off inefficiently and benefiting the better off more efficiently.

Likewise, utilitarians account for the moral imperative to respect people's autonomous choices by arguing that such respect normally lets people maximize their well-being. Hence, respecting autonomy is utility maximizing. Although that is often the case, we can easily imagine cases in which respecting individual autonomy does not maximize utility. This is the case whenever someone is not good at calculating his own welfare. Nevertheless, since sophisticated utilitarianism is able to account for many of the moral judgments made by nonutilitarians, the behavioral judgments of utilitarians do not always look that different from more complex multiprinciple theories.

Libertarianism A similar analysis can be provided for another single-principle theory. In the current standard language, the libertarian ethic is based only on the principle of respect for autonomy. Nevertheless, libertarianism can account for many moral judgments that square with utilitarian and multiprinciple theories. Often (but clearly not always) letting people make their own choices by respecting their autonomy will do more good than violating it. Libertarians may end up maximizing the good produced by setting out to respect autonomy while utilitarians may end up respecting autonomy by setting out to maximize utility. The interesting cases, of course, are the special ones where these relations do not correlate.

Edmund Pellegrino's Beneficence-in-Trust Another sophisticated single-principle theory is defended by physician-ethicist Edmund Pellegrino, the former president of Catholic University, chair of the US President's Council on Bioethics, and my predecessor as director of the Kennedy Institute of Ethics. He claims that his medical ethics is built on a single principle, what he calls "beneficence-in-trust."[6] It has similarities to Hippocratic theory in having the health professional commit "in-trust" to benefit the patient, but his unique theory of the patient's good makes his position much more plausible than and different from Hippocratic ethics. He holds that there are four levels of the patient's good, the biomedical good being the lowest. He calls the second level "the patient's best interest," by which he means the patient's concept of his own good as the patient perceives it subjectively. The third level is the "good of the patient as a human person," referring to the human's capacity to reason. Finally, the highest element of the good is "the last or ultimate good," the "telos of human life," as it is perceived by the patient.[7] Moreover, Pellegrino can capture many of the concerns for the worst off that usually would fall under the principle of justice by incorporating the Catholic social concept of the common good.[8]

Hippocratic Beneficence By contrast, the single principle in Hippocratic ethics requires that the physician benefit the patient according to the physician's ability and judgment, and that the physician protect the patient from harm. It is a truly unique ethical principle. It combines beneficence and nonmaleficence into a single principle the way utilitarianism does, but it limits the relevant benefit to the good of the patient and assesses that benefit paternalistically, "according to the physician's ability and judgment." Contrary to the pop culture of physicians, it gives no priority to not harming as the modern slogan "primum non nocere" implies. It is hard to imagine that any theorist other than one working in a professional setting would have opted for this form of a single-principle theory. Certainly, no normative theory in biomedical ethics opts for this rather odd form of a single-principle theory.

❧

It is plausible to view these single-principle theories as corrupt accounts of the data from the common morality offered by fallible humans who do the best they can to capture the moral norms. Clever utilitarians and beneficence-in-trust formulations do a good job of providing an account that squares with our considered moral judgments much of the time, even if they have a very difficult time accounting for the tough cases—when maximizing utility requires violating individual autonomy, when the patient's ultimate well-being can only be served by compromising other aspects of the patient's good, or when justice requires targeting patients who can only be helped inefficiently.

Tristram Engelhardt's Two-Principle Theory

The philosopher-physician H. Tristram Engelhardt is an example of a physician who makes no pretense of offering a professionally generated ethic. Influenced by Hegel and the libertarian philosopher Robert Nozick, Engelhardt affirms the principle of permission (what in his first edition was the principle of autonomy) as the first principle.[9] He is one who denies the possibility of what he calls the monotheistic solution—the use of reason or intuition to gain knowledge of a single set of norms that make up a common morality. At least outside of his religious perspective (discussed in chapter 5), he believes that, aside from the principle of permission or autonomy, there is no account of a single, universal morality that is persuasive. Thus, for him, the principle of permission requires that real people actually give their consent to be governed by a moral system. Since no rational or moral sense provides a single common framework, Engelhardt makes all social interaction rest morally on the permission of the individual. Only within the communities generated by the granting of such permission is there a norm of beneficence. For Engelhardt, no principle of justice exists calling for distribution of resources according to some preconceived pattern (such as distribution according to need).[10] Thus, Engelhardt's two principles operating within communities created through actual personal commitments produce an ethic far from the traditional professional ethic but one that is also distant from the view that most contemporary theorists associate with the common morality. Nevertheless, he is quite capable of accounting for most considered moral judgments relying on his principles of permission and beneficence.

Baruch Brody's Five Conflicting Appeals

Having already explored the *Belmont Report*'s three principles and the four principles of Beauchamp and Childress, we can next consider Rice philosopher Baruch Brody's normative theory, which he refers to as "five conflicting appeals."[11] In table 7.1, I number them as he ordered them in his book. He is one of the theorists who do not use the language of principles. Rather he speaks of normative criteria as "appeals." Still, at least some of his appeals are functionally like principles. He claims these five appeals must be balanced against one another. The list adds complexities.

One of his appeals, for example, is to the virtues.[12] One can imagine balancing several principles of right action against one another, but it seems difficult to imagine how one would balance principles against an appeal to the virtues. Principles of right action identify characteristics of actions. One can determine simply by assessing the action whether it produces benefit, respects autonomy, or distributes a good according to some predetermined pattern of justice. The virtues, however, refer to character traits of actors—the will to do good, the manifesting of courage or love, or the showing of compassion. These cannot be assessed independent of the person involved whose character traits are of concern.

Since virtues refer to the character of an actor and not the characteristics of an action, it is hard to see how they could conflict with action principles. One either benefits the patient or does not, independent of whether the actor manifests some character trait such as compassion or even benevolence. One may benefit the patient without compassion (if one is acting impeccably in order to gain a promotion, for example) or one can act compassionately but choose the wrong action and thus fail to benefit the patient. There seems to be no way that compassion, one of the most fashionable virtues in medicine, could "conflict" with producing benefit for a patient.

Nevertheless, some of the other appeals of Brody clearly can come in conflict. His first appeal is to consequences, and his third is to respect for persons.[13] Here he is merely replicating the classical conflict between consequentialist and deontological normative theories. His position is that, when the two conflict, they must be balanced, a position similar to that of Beauchamp and Childress.

Brody's list looks quite different from the standard four-principle list. It is a list of appeals rather than a list of principles. It cites consequences rather than beneficence and nonmaleficence, but this would seem to be essentially the same appeal, subject to the linguistic variations that will be inevitable when theorists codify the insights of the common morality. He does not include respect for autonomy, but, as with the *Belmont Report*, he includes respect for persons, which covers very similar territory. He resists the metaphor of using scales to "weigh" conflicting claims that sometimes come with the four-principle theorists, but this is merely to make the point that the appeals cannot be quantified.[14]

Brody's list of five appeals also includes an "appeal to rights," which he places second on his list.[15] As far as I can tell, what he thinks of as a right is no more than the reciprocal of the duties that follow from respect for persons, his third appeal. For example, if respect for persons calls for a physician to respect autonomy by getting informed consent, that same concept can be expressed as the patient having a right to consent before being treated. If this is correct, Brody's second and third appeals are redundant. That may be a problem if, in the balancing, the same notion (such as getting consent) counts twice, giving it double consideration.

A similar problem arises with Brody's fifth appeal, "cost-effectiveness and justice."[16] These seem to be placeholders for the moral insight that the social dimensions of one's actions count. Justice is surely an independent moral appeal, a separate principle in the schemes of many normative theorists, including Beauchamp and Childress. Justice could already be accounted for in the duties derived from Brody's appeal to respect for persons, but some would count justice as a separate principle, in which case it is correctly considered a separate "appeal." Cost-effectiveness, however, seems to be an appeal to producing as much good consequences as possible per unit of resources. If this is what is implied, it is an appeal that is not only different from justice but also redundant with Brody's appeal to consequences, an appeal already accounted for. Once again, appealing separately to consequences and to cost-effectiveness may run the risk of double counting the same moral consideration.

In the end, Brody's normative theory is within shouting distance of the four principles. If one separates out the virtues as not properly part of a theory of right action, we are left with appeals to consequences and cost-effectiveness (beneficence and nonmaleficence), respect for persons (including respect for autonomy and other duty-based principles), and justice—rather like the Beauchamp and Childress list. It is surely within the variations that one would expect with the necessarily arbitrary choices of language and emphasis that comes with theorizing. After one makes adjustments for what seem like minor problems (such as attempting to balance action criteria against virtues), the Brody norms are more or less compatible with the *Belmont* and four-principle theories.

W. D. Ross's Six Prima Facie Duties

Another normative theory of ethics that attempts to systematize our intuitions about moral requiredness is in many ways the progenitor of all the other theories. W. D. Ross, another previous Gifford lecturer, puts forward a list of right-making characteristics that he calls "prima facie duties" in his famous work *The Right and the Good*.[17] He explicitly numbers them, making clear that he has six in mind.[18] They include beneficence, nonmaleficence, and justice, as do many of the previous theories we have surveyed. To these he adds duties growing out of previous acts of one's own, mentioning duties of fidelity (promise-keeping and veracity as well as duties of reparation) and duties growing out of previous acts of others, what he calls duties of gratitude. None of these show up explicitly on any previous lists we have considered, but they all might be seen as explications of the notion of respect for persons.

Two puzzles arise with Ross's list. First, he considers the duty of self-improvement to differ from the duty of beneficence, based on the view that beneficence calls for benefits to others, apparently in the form of pleasure. Others would collapse the duty of self-improvement with more general duties of beneficence. Second, and most puzzling, he includes no duty to respect autonomy. Perhaps like some other theorists he believes the duty to let others be self-determining can be derived from the other principles. Perhaps it is simply an omission that we can attribute to the fact that no finite theorist gets things exactly right. Surely, however, for more recent ethical theorists working in biomedical ethics, the omission of any consideration of autonomy or self-determination remains a puzzle.

My Seven- (or Nine-) Principle Theory

Having considered all the available normative lists of principles or equivalent, including heavy exposure to Ross and some exposure to the first edition of Beauchamp and Childress, I set out to attempt my first normative theory construction in the late 1970s, feeling compelled to make yet another set of modifications.[19] Two adjustments and one additional qualification seemed necessary.

Unpacking Respect for Persons First, I was not satisfied with limiting respect for persons to autonomy. I preferred the more inclusive language of the *Belmont Report* (while not accepting their controversial and apparently mistaken attempt to place protection of the welfare of children under the "respect for persons" notion). I expanded the general notion of respect for persons so that it included, in addition to respecting autonomy, also showing respect by considering the Rossian duties of fidelity and veracity (what he called duties growing out of previous acts of one's own). Influenced by Kantian consideration of the maxim prohibiting of killing of humans, I also claimed that showing respect for persons would require a prima facie duty not to kill them. I wanted this formulated so that it would not require doing everything to preserve life, no matter the uselessness or burden involved, so I included a principle of avoidance of killing in my list of the principles that were not designed to maximize good consequences. The substantive importance of this addition is that there is an independent principle that avoiding killing is right-making of actions, a position that differs from utilitarians who derive the general prohibition against killing from the principle of utility and thus expose themselves to the possibility that killing would be acceptable if only it does more good than harm. The utilitarian's only response to the accusation that killing would automatically be acceptable whenever it did as much or more good compared with the harm it would do would be an appeal to long-term or rule utility, such as is seen in Beauchamp.[20]

With these adjustments, my normative theory includes what can be counted as seven principles: beneficence, nonmaleficence, justice, fidelity, veracity, (respect for) autonomy, and avoidance of killing. I have tried to make clear that the apparent additions of fidelity, veracity, and avoidance of killing were merely my explication of what I understood a full theory of respect for persons to require, not a substantive change from earlier lists.

I acknowledge that treating avoidance of killing as a separate, freestanding, prima facie principle may lead to different conclusions from colleagues who would ground a duty not to kill humans in utility or in nonmaleficence, as Beauchamp and Childress and Gert's group do. I want to claim that killing people normally harms them; this alone explains most cases in which it is wrong to kill. I want to say something else, however. I want to claim that there is something prima facie wrong with the killing of a human, even in the rare case when it does not harm them, that is, does not set back their interests. This could include cases in which the person is permanently unconscious and can be said no longer to have interests.[21] It could also include cases in which the person is rationally suicidal and claims he or she would not be harmed by being killed.

I acknowledge that not everyone accepts the notion that killing others has an intrinsic wrongness to it as well as normally harming the one who is killed. This additional feature of killing at least provides a basis for explaining the traditional received moral judgments that euthanasia, merciful killing of another upon that person's request, and suicide are morally suspect even if they do not harm the one killed. Either I am mistaken in finding this intrinsic wrongness of killing in the common morality, or others are wrong in failing to see it there. If I am wrong, I have a great deal of company.

If I am permitted to differentiate respect for persons into four component principles—fidelity, autonomy, veracity, and avoidance of killing—then, along with beneficence, nonmaleficence, and justice, I end up with a seven-principle normative theory. The similarity with the other theories that differentiate principles somewhat differently should be apparent, however. I would have no objection to claiming that my four principles subsumed under "respect for persons" are really subprinciples of the more general "respect for persons" principle.

Differentiating Hippocratic and Social Utility   The second major adjustment I have made in my list of normative ethical principles is the differentiation of beneficence and nonmaleficence into two components: Hippocratic and social versions of these principles. I have noted that traditional Hippocratic ethics shares with classical social utilitarianism a commitment to the two principles beneficence and nonmaleficence. Both find it necessary to integrate judgments of benefit and harm into a single metric, by subtracting anticipated harm from anticipated benefit, á la Bentham, by calculating the ratio of benefit to harm expected from

alternative courses of action, or by ranking nonmaleficence over beneficence as the nineteenth-century purveyor of the "primum non nocere"
slogan and W. D. Ross were apparently inclined to do.[22]

There is, however, a critical difference between Hippocratic and classical utility. Classical utilitarianism insists on estimating expected net
benefit for each person affected by an action and summing or otherwise
combining the individual estimates. Hippocratic utility, on the other
hand, militantly insists that only benefit and harm to the patient count.
The physician is to benefit the patient and protect the patient from harm.
It is commonly added that considering the impacts of one's actions on
other parties is not morally relevant—indeed, is specifically prohibited.

Thus, I note that, although I have put forward seven principles, some
will apply them at the level of the individual, others at the social level.
Clinical medical ethics have historically limited the clinician's moral
horizon to the level of interaction with the individual patient. Problems
of social utility maximizing were off the table, as were problems of justice. Hence, the absence of any theory of justice in classical Hippocratic
ethics can be understood if not accepted.

Two More Possible Principles   I need to make clear that I am not
locked into a list of seven principles. Hence, I need to make one final
qualification. I concur in principle with Ross's addition of duties of reparation and gratitude but note that usually these do not come into play in
most medical ethical controversy. They would, however, in a case in
which a physician had, perhaps by accident, harmed a patient and felt a
special duty to benefit that patient as compensation over and above the
duties of beneficence that the physician would have to the patient. Thus,
it seems to make sense that a physician forced to choose between two
patients who could be benefited equally would opt to benefit the one
needing help because the physician had previously caused an injury.

Similarly, a society might have duties of reparation that could have an
impact on the allocation of its health care resources. A city that had
discriminated seriously on racial grounds and that was later deciding how
to distribute health clinics in the city might consider it prima facie its

obligation to target those areas with populations suffering from poor health because of the city's prior discrimination. It might even consider it morally required to give those portions of the city clinic resources beyond what would be provided to other portions of the city with patients who were equally poorly off but had not suffered the effects of the city's discrimination. Duties of reparation as well as duties of gratitude are relevant in principle, even if normally they do not come into play in health care ethics. If these are added, it could be said that I favor a nine-principle theory.

The differences between my list of seven or nine principles and other lists, while occasionally leading to different moral judgments, are at most differences at the margins. I still present a list that resembles the others in most critical respects. Insofar as we are all looking at pretheoretical moral insights in the common morality, it is not surprising that they are similar. For one who accepts the common grounding of normative moral judgments accessible to all reasonable or serious people in and out of the professions, this should not be surprising. For one who accepts human finitude and the necessity of arbitrary linguistic conventions, it should not be surprising that modest differences occur. Perhaps if we could all gather together and attempt to replicate ideal observers these differences would disappear. Nevertheless, in a postmodern world that recognizes a "value-dependent realism" in which multiple linguistically different accounts of reality are not only possible but inevitable, our descriptions of the common morality that get incorporated into normative ethical theory will continue to reveal somewhat different descriptions even if we are describing the same moral reality. The fact that ethical theorists, like the rest of us, are finite, fallible humans makes it even more likely that normative theories will manifest marginal differences.

Gert's Ten Rules: A Single Principle in Disguise?

Not having identified any plausible theory that happens to have a list of eight principles, I turn finally to the ten rules of Gert, Culver, Clouser, and others associated with the Dartmouth group. They place considerable emphasis on their claim that they are not principlists.[23] They offer, instead, ten moral rules.[24]

Their attack on the use of principles, however, is really an attack on the claim that no overarching method exists for resolving conflict among principles, that they must be balanced intuitively. That, in fact, is the view of Beauchamp and Childress and others including Brody, but that is not an inherent characteristic of principles. The single-principle theories, for example, do not require intuitive balancing among principles (although they do require some method—perhaps intuition—for determining which actions are utility or autonomy maximizing).

Some principlists, myself included, do support some limited strategies for resolving at least some conflicts among principles.[25] John Rawls is an example of a prominent theorist who makes use of the concept of principles—the principle of justice, in particular—and has a clear ranking of one principle over another, justice over utility and the first principle of justice over the second.[26] I see no reason why the Dartmouth team's account of the common morality need eschew the language of principles as long as that terminology is dissociated from the claim that necessarily there can be no method for resolving any conflicts among principles except intuitive balancing.

In fact, if one looks at the ten rules proposed by the Dartmouth group, they have the look and feel of principles even if they persist in calling them rules. "Rules" is a term usually reserved for more specific moral injunctions, the kind that often show up in codes of ethics, whereas "principles" refers to more general, abstract, right-making characteristics of action. For example, it might be said that "Always get consent before surgery" is a rule derived mainly from the principle of autonomy (but perhaps also from beneficence).

Considering the ten rules of the Dartmouth group, most do not have the normal specificity of rules. They are essentially as abstract as principles and can be seen as surrogates for principles. "Do not deprive of freedom" is closely associated with what principle-based theories would call the principle of respect for autonomy. "Do not break your promise" is the functional equivalent of my principle of promise-keeping or fidelity. "Do not deceive" is the equivalent of my principle of veracity. "Do not kill" is the equivalent of my principle of avoiding killing. Several of their other rules are clearly derived from what I would call the principle of nonmaleficence. These include "do not cause pain," "do not disable," and "do not deprive of pleasure."

In fact, Gert and his colleagues frequently affirm that all their rules are designed to avoid, prevent, or remove harms. It would be consistent with their theory to claim that they have a one-principle theory and that the principle is nonmaleficence.[27] Their ten rules would then be seen as derivative from their one principle.

Only the last three of their rules are harder to map on standard lists of principles. These include "do not cheat," which probably can be understood as related to my principles of fidelity and veracity; "do not break the law," which seems related to commitments made that one must keep in order to avoid infidelity; and "do not neglect your duty," a concept that Gert and colleagues use in a technical sense of fulfilling obligations related to special roles, such as the role of health professional. That also seems related to promises made, such as the promises made at the time of licensure or oath taking.

My point is that each of the Dartmouth group's ten rules can be seen as functionally related to one or more of the principles of some other normative theories. Moreover, these Dartmouth authors themselves acknowledge that they see all the rules as related to the moral requirement not to cause harm. They specifically say of the moral rules that their "essential role is to proscribe actions that commonly cause harm."[28] A bit later in the same volume they claim, "the point of morality is the lessening of the amount of evil or harm suffered by those protected by morality."[29] Nothing would be changed if we recoded the Dartmouth team's theory to say that it is a single-principle theory based on nonmaleficence in which the general principle of not harming is further specified or elucidated by ten moral rules. This would make their theory one of a group of single-principle theories in which, in their case, they try to support all the moral insights available in the common morality by the single principle of nonmaleficence. They would still be left with a problem analogous to the other single-principle theories (such as utilitarianism and libertarianism) of accounting for our moral duties, such as respect for autonomy by deriving them from nonmaleficence.

The result of the Dartmouth group's scheme is some contortions to try to fit all the insights of the common morality into the container of nonmaleficence. As with the other single-principle theories, they find themselves dropping some moral insights commonly incorporated into a moral framework. The most conspicuous is the principle of justice, taken as a principle calling for a morally right end-state pattern of the distribution of the good. Justice for them is merely a synonym for doing the right thing by following the rules.[30] Engelhardt also drops justice, and the utilitarians squeeze it into their theory by claiming that decreasing marginal utility often makes it utility maximizing to distribute resources to the person who has the least, a claim that often—but not always—works to give priority to the worst off.

Most unusual in the Dartmouth group's normative scheme is the absence of a "principle" or rule to identify the production of good as prima facie right-making. Almost all other theories include beneficence as a principle of right action. The Dartmouth group claims that doing good is not a requirement of the moral rules. It may be a moral ideal but not a rule.[31]

In the end, the Dartmouth group's scheme of moral rules that starts out sounding so antithetical to principle-based approaches ends up sounding more and more like a single-principle theory based on nonmaleficence in which many of the standard principles such as autonomy, veracity, fidelity, and avoidance of killing (and perhaps even justice) can be derived. Surely this ten-rule system, which incorporates the moral notions that others would call principles, differs in critical respects—the lack of any independent basis for justice, autonomy, and other moral norms, the unusual handling of beneficence, and the rejection of balancing strategies for resolving conflict. Nevertheless, it is not unrealistic to note that, as an attempt to systematize a theoretical account of the pretheoretical common morality, their system has distinct parallels with the other normative theories available and would lead to the same moral conclusions most of the time.

It is reasonable to conclude that, among the normative theories in biomedical ethics that are derivable from natural methods such as reason and experience, the differences are relatively minor—minor enough to be explained by the limited perspectives of the various theorists and the necessity of arbitrarily choosing a language for describing what can be called the common morality.

The Criteria for an Acceptable Public Ethic for the Professions

This suggests that the theorists who attempt to codify the moral insights that are generally available and known to reasonable or serious people have developed a set of norms—usually called principles, but sometimes called prima facie duties, rules, or appeals—that come close to organizing our moral experience in ways that account for most moral judgments that are widely shared. When moral norms conflict, there will be differences in interpretation and priority based on cultural, religious, and other social variables. Nevertheless, most religious people who understand morality to have a religious basis and most secular people who understand the basis differently will come out agreeing on most moral judgments most of the time. That is what one would expect from people who share public, natural, verifiable ways of knowing morality.

Differences occur because humans are fallible animals. They perceive the moral reality from a finite perspective. Their reasoning is inevitably flawed. They will necessarily be prone to error and make mistakes. Most critically, cultural biases and value commitments will distort judgments, especially in new and controversial areas. Nevertheless, the participants in the theory-constructing process who rely on these shared methods of moral knowledge produce normative theories that are within shouting distance.

It might be, however, that the contributors to the process of theory formation share enough Western philosophical and religious premises that they share the same biases. It is the nature of the epistemologies that rely on standard devices—social contracts, ideal observer theories, reasoning about the natural law, moral sense theories, and other natural means of knowing—that accuracy comes from elimination of biases that might be introduced by working from a limited perspective. It is useful to see if there could be more public, less academic devices for producing a set of moral norms for the professions.

The ideal way of generating an ethic for a profession such as medicine would be to first have a public discussion from which the basic norms for society are articulated and then, based on those norms, have members of a profession and laypeople jointly agree on the norms for lay–professional relations. In 1981, when I wrote *A Theory of Medical Ethics*, no such effort had been attempted, so I had to propose my own version of what a commonly agreed-upon set of norms might look like. Referring to this as the first of a three-part social contract, I had to imagine the criteria for the ideal group of citizens of the world meeting to identify such a set of norms including:

- All parties of the world community would participate, directly or indirectly, in establishing a set of norms.
- They would try to act as if they did not know where they were in the social order and did not know their particular interests or abilities.
- They would nevertheless strive to have maximum information about the social, psychological, economic, medical, and other general facts of the human community.
- They would attempt to replicate all the other characteristics of ideal observers, including being disinterested, dispassionate, consistent, and normal in all other respects.

It is from this hypothetical exercise that I identified my seven principles (beneficence, nonmaleficence, autonomy, fidelity, veracity, avoidance of killing, and justice). Once that exercise was completed, I moved on to a second contract—an agreement between laypeople and health professionals about the moral rules governing lay–professional relations.

Still working in a hypothetical mode, I imagined people at the table with the following characteristics:

- Both laypeople and professionals would have their voices fairly represented.
- They would be expected to create a set of moral norms for the roles of health professional and health layperson while having their conduct constrained by the general norms of the first contract.
- They would leave the maximum possible space for individual professionals and individual laypeople to be free to establish more concrete agreements for the terms of the relations between specific patients and providers.

On this basis I proposed a social contract—I called it a "Draft Medical Ethical Covenant"—an agreement between health professionals and the lay community articulating the ethical norms for their interactions. It included the principles I have described here: fidelity, autonomy, veracity, avoidance of killing, and justice. Within these prior constraints I recognized the moral mandate of striving to do good for one another and protect from harm. It was an attempt to affirm that both laypeople and professionals were active moral agents with rights and responsibilities. It made clear that health professionals gain special rights and responsibilities from the citizenry and are accountable to them for their conduct.

Since then, several public efforts to hold such meetings to articulate codifications of the duties of health professionals and laypeople have actually occurred. I have been pleased that the codes that have emerged have been rather close to the contract I imagined in the 1980s. I remain convinced that my seven-principle form of a basic theory of morally right action is a good—dare I say, the best—way of describing the norms widely shared, at least one defensible account of the common morality. I acknowledge that other accounts are also plausible—that they use different language to provide another accurate description of the underlying moral reality. It is good, however, to have available publicly created descriptions as well, so, in closing this volume, I discuss two such accounts and highlight remaining differences that need attention.

The Council on Europe Convention for Protection of Human Rights and Dignity of the Human Being with Regard to the Application of Biology and Biomedicine: Convention on Human Rights and Biomedicine

The first effort that could possibly be said to be an attempt to conform to these criteria at the level of specifying norms for professional and lay conduct in the biomedical arena was the Council of Europe's Convention for Protection of Human Rights and Dignity of the Human Being with Regard to the Application of Biology and Biomedicine, commonly referred to by its subtitle, the Convention on Human Rights and Biomedicine, or simply the Bioethics Convention. Twenty-one of the forty member nations signed on immediately to this convention. It is the first international, legally binding set of norms that addressed bioethical issues such as human subjects research, genetics, embryology, and transplantation. It also addresses matters of human dignity in the practice of medicine, equitable access to health care, and informed consent.

While this is a convention dealing with the area of biomedical ethics, it specifically acknowledges the background commitment to the United Nations General Assembly's Universal Declaration of Human Rights adopted December 10, 1948, as well as other international agreements that extent beyond the European context. The first chapter of the convention outlines what are called "general provisions." These are as close as the document comes to what others would call general principles. If these were compared to the lists of principles coming from the theorists that we have already discussed, there would be, with some stretching, a partial fit.

The first article commits member states to "protect the dignity and identity of all human beings and guarantee everyone, without discrimination, respect for their integrity and other rights and fundamental freedoms with regard to the application of biology and medicine." The term so prevalent in European ethics documents—dignity—is given pride of first place in the presentation. It is connected to the notions of rights and fundamental freedoms, thus confirming my suggestion that dignity is possibly an alternate way of affirming respect for persons and the rights associated with such respect.

The text next commits to the primacy of the human being, saying that the "interests and welfare of the human being shall prevail over the sole interest of society or science." This may reflect a lingering Hippocratic notion of the central focus on the individual at the expense of matters of the common good or social justice.

The third article explicitly introduces equitable access to health care of appropriate quality. This is followed with an anomalous commitment that "any intervention in the health field, including research, must be carried out in accordance with relevant professional obligations and standards." As we have seen, this is an ambiguous and potentially confusing commitment. It could mean that professionally generated or articulated norms from, for example, national medical associations should always apply. If this is the meaning, then the Council of Europe is making the strange—indeed, irrational—commitment that it will blindly accept norms chosen by professional groups even if those norms directly affect the laypeople upon whom they have impact, and even if the lay public rejects those norms. We have seen many examples of ethical topics about which the professionally generated norm is in conflict with what laypeople believe should count as proper ethical behavior by professionals.

For example, the profession has at various times adopted norms governing truth-telling to dying patients, standards for informed consent, policies on professional advertising, confidentiality rules, health care rationing standards, and positions on providing nutrition and hydration to patients that conflict with the views of laypeople, governments, and religious groups. On the other hand, the Council of Europe may simply be committing itself here to acting in accord with standards for professional behavior adopted by more legitimate authorities, whether they be governmental, philosophical, or religious. On its face, there is no way of knowing what counts as a "relevant" professional obligation or standard.

The Council of Europe Bioethics Convention then goes on in additional chapters to put forward more specific rules governing consent, access to information, the human genome, scientific research, organ transplant, and trafficking in human bodies. The fact that the Council feels comfortable speaking normatively on these concrete issues and promulgating rules of conduct related to them suggests that it cannot any longer believe that the professional bodies have custody of these norms. Presumably, this European supernational body is claiming moral authority for the citizens of its member states whether they be lay or members of the health professions.

The real problem with the Council of Europe's Bioethics Convention is that it, at best, claims to speak for the twenty-one or so countries of Europe that are signatories. It is thus open to claims of parochialism, of not speaking for most of the people of the world. Even if the convention represents a shift in moral authority away from the professional groups in the direction of a more eclectic collection of lay and professional perspectives, it is still a parochial perspective if one considers the Asian, African, and new world countries who are not at the table. Something even broader is needed.

Universal Declaration on Human Rights and Its Application to Bioethics

For some time, one publicly generated moral document has been available at the level of what I have called the first social contract. That document is the Universal Declaration of Human Rights.

The Universal Declaration of Human Rights

In 1948 the United Nations General Assembly adopted without opposition a declaration clarifying the UN Charter's affirmation of "fundamental human rights, and dignity and worth of the human person." The product of the UN's Commission on Human Rights, the declaration is the first global affirmation of human rights from a public body with worldwide standing. That declaration provides the background for the Universal Declaration on Bioethics and Human Rights.

Universal Declaration on Bioethics and Human Rights

Until 2005, no comparable document existed internationally that addressed specifically the area of biomedical ethics. Professional groups had produced countless codes of ethics, but they normally were produced exclusively by members of the profession involved. Sometimes they were not even disclosed to the public. The Hippocratic Oath contains within it a commitment to keep knowledge of medicine secret. In the nineteenth century, the Kappa Lambda Society was itself secret and its so-called Hippocratic code of ethics was not made known to any patients or even to physicians who were not members of the society. As recently as 1970, the British Medical Association refused to disclose to the public the code of ethics that it had promulgated for its members. To this day, national medical associations, such as the American Medical Association, produce unilateral codes of ethics in which a committee made up exclusively of members of the association writes a version of a code that is then adopted by the association without any formal input from members of the public, religious leaders, or other opinion leaders who might have different perspectives on the ethics of the lay–professional relation. This unilateral, professionally generated code is then bestowed (or inflicted) on the public.

Occasionally, international professional bodies such as the World Medical Association have spoken, as in 1948, when it first promulgated the modern paraphrase of the Hippocratic Oath known as the Declaration of Geneva. Still, only members of the profession have even indirect representation in the process. The vast majority of the world's citizens—medical laypeople—have no voice in the group's code-writing activities.

Religious groups have also promulgated statements on the ethics of the practice of the professions including the health professions. Sometimes their role is premised on the claim that the critical moral knowledge is revealed through channels within the religious organization—its scriptures, tradition, and authoritative teachers. In other cases, even if the religious group accepts in principle the role of natural means of knowing—reasoning about the natural law, for example—still outsiders have played little or no role in the generation of the codes of ethics and moral stances adopted by religious bodies. It is sometimes ambiguous whether the religiously generated positions are meant to apply only to professional practitioners who are part of that religious group or are to apply to all practicing the profession, even if they are not associated with the religious tradition involved. Presumably, practitioners and patients outside that tradition would have little reason to give the pronouncements serious attention, just as laypeople and health professionals outside organized national and international medical organizations have no reason to accept guidance by professionally generated codifications. Academics have written treatises that strive to rely on reason and experience, claiming that their suggested codifications should be accepted by all parties in the professional–lay interaction, but often these have lacked any legitimacy and authority beyond the sheer force of the academic's powers of persuasion.

In 2005, something unique in the history of professional ethics occurred. A public international body, the United Nations Educational, Scientific, and Cultural Organization (UNESCO), working with its International Bioethics Committee (IBC) and its Inter-Governmental Bioethics Committee (IGBC), produced a bioethical codification that it called the Universal Declaration on Bioethics and Human Rights (UDBHR). It was adopted by acclamation by the member countries of UNESCO on October 19, 2005.

The process is unique in the history of bioethics. The IBC, which took responsibility for much of the drafting, was made up of thirty-six people from member countries. Appointed by the director-general of UNESCO, a substantial majority are apparently medical laypeople—philosophers, lawyers, and government officials.[32]

A UN interagency committee met in 2004 to ensure improved coordination of activities and thinking on bioethics throughout the United Nations system. It included participants from FAO, UNESCO, UNU,

WHO, WIPO ALESCO, the European Commission, the Council of Europe, OECD, and the WTO. In August of 2004 the IBC heard from representatives from religious/spiritual perspectives including Confucianism, Judaism, Hinduism, Islam, Buddhism, and Catholicism. The result is the first truly international, representative codification of norms for bioethics that the world has ever seen. Rather than reflecting the norms of the professional groups or national, religious, or ideological bodies, the Universal Declaration can legitimately claim to speak for virtually all citizens of the world (at least through the representatives working on their behalf). No matter how flawed the final content of this document may be (and its problems seem minor), this is a first in the history of applied ethics.

The UDBHR Principles

The UDBHR specifically acknowledges the Universal Declaration of Human Rights as one of its foundational premises. It then spells out in twenty-eight articles a list of rights that are meant to govern the practice of medicine and related practices in bioethics. The central themes of bioethicists' normative theory are well represented.

Article 4 specifies that direct and indirect benefits to patients, research participants, and other affected individuals should be maximized, and harms should be minimized. In philosophical jargon, the principles of beneficence and nonmaleficence are affirmed, including a recognition that these principles are relevant beyond the Hippocratic focus on the individual patient.

Articles 5–7 explicitly acknowledge that the autonomy of persons to make decisions is to be respected. In philosophical terms, respect for autonomy is affirmed. This is further spelled out in Articles 6 and 7 as it applies to autonomous persons and those lacking capacity to consent.

Several articles (including articles 8, 10, and 11) address issues that most ethicists would classify under the rubric of the principle of justice. Article 8 is titled "Equality, Justice, and Equity," categories sorely lacking in the Hippocratic Oath and many other professional codes as well as in certain sets of normative principles or rules by certain academics.[33] The fundamental equality of all human beings is acknowledged, and discrimination and stigmatization are condemned. Respect for the vulnerable is enjoined.

Article 9 commits to privacy and confidentiality "to the extent possible," provided that it is consistent with international law and, in particular, human rights law. It is debatable whether that is consistent with recent British and American provisions that require disclosure of confidential information when necessary to protect others from the credible threat of grave bodily harm. There is at least recognition of the ethical requirement of confidentiality that is not to be overridden on paternalistic grounds that were seen in many older professionally generated codes.

Several articles focus on additional principles of social ethics beyond what is required by the commitment to equality, justice, and equity. Article 13 affirms social solidarity; article 14, social responsibility for health; article 15, the necessity of sharing the fruits of medical research. Article 16 extends the agenda to future generations, and article 17 embraces the environment and biosphere.

This is a remarkably refreshing and thorough first try at a public international codification that grounds an ethic for laypeople and professionals in shared moral insights accessible to all human beings rather than professionally generated codes imposed on patients often without them even knowing it. It is not as clear on what I called the principle of avoiding killing as it applies to medicine. Probably no international consensus could be crafted in that area. Some of the most divisive issues—abortion, euthanasia, stem cells, genetics, and organ transplantation—are not confronted, perhaps because they are too specific, but more likely because they were too controversial and could not generate consensus.

Finally, the document is not clear on what should happen should the various principles articulated come into conflict with one another. We are told that these moral considerations are grounded in human rights. Human rights are often seen as "trumping," as requiring full conformity regardless of conflicting norms. We are told that "human rights and fundamental freedoms are to be fully respected," a pretty bold statement.

Yet we are also told in article 26 that "this Declaration is to be understood as a whole and the principles are to be understood as complementary and interrelated. Each principle is to be considered in the context of the other principles, as appropriate and relevant in the circumstances."

That may give too much wiggle room and may conflict with the bold commitment to full respect for human rights and fundamental freedoms. To theorists who call for more than a vague intuitive balancing of competing claims as well as those who in Kantian fashion affirm maxims as imperatives without exception, too many ambiguities may remain. This first attempt at a universal public declaration on bioethics and human rights reflects the convergence of the natural epistemologies of religious ethical systems with secular ethics that has given rise to a substantial consensus of a list of principles, duties, rules, or rights affirmed by all reasonable people serious about ethical matters and that is manifest in the various theories of biomedical ethics.

Proper understanding of the affirmation of human freedom and autonomy suggests substantial room for sectarian medical practices among those groups of laypeople and professionals who share additional moral imperatives that they believe are known to them via supernatural means of revelation. As long as those do not conflict with the rights and freedoms expressed in the broader universal statements, such imperatives should not be a problem. This convergence of religious and secular moral systems constrained by our awareness of human finitude so that individual patients and providers are given maximum freedom to pursue their own understanding of what morality requires represents an enormous advance for society in its understanding of professional ethics as it relates to laypeople. It is surely a vast advance over the day when professional groups claimed the authority to articulate and generate codes of ethics that could be imposed on laypeople without their knowledge of consent.

The contrast with more traditional medical ethics grounded in professional sources of knowledge and religious revelation is dramatic. Patients of the world will be patient no longer. They finally claim their place as full and equal active partners in the process of formulating an ethic for their relations with professionals.

APPENDIX

UNIVERSAL DECLARATION ON BIOETHICS AND HUMAN RIGHTS

The General Conference, . . .
Proclaims the principles that follow and *adopts* the present Declaration.

General Provisions

Article 1—Scope

1. This Declaration addresses ethical issues related to medicine, life sciences and associated technologies as applied to human beings, taking into account their social, legal and environmental dimensions.
2. This Declaration is addressed to States. As appropriate and relevant, it also provides guidance to decisions or practices of individuals, groups, communities, institutions and corporations, public and private.

Article 2—Aims

The aims of this Declaration are:
  (a) to provide a universal framework of principles and procedures to guide States in the formulation of their legislation, policies or other instrument in the field of bioethics;
  (b) to guide the actions of individuals, groups, communities, institutions and corporations, public and private;

193

(c) to promote respect for human dignity and protect human rights, by ensuring respect for the life of human beings, and fundamental freedoms, consistent with international human rights law;

(d) to recognize the importance of freedom of scientific research and the benefits derived from scientific and technological developments, while stressing the need for such research and developments to occur within the framework of ethical principles set out in this Declaration and to respect human dignity, human rights and fundamental freedoms;

(e) to foster multidisciplinary and pluralistic dialogue about bioethical issues between all stakeholders and within society as a whole;

(f) to promote equitable access to medical, scientific and technological developments as well as the greatest possible flow and the rapid sharing of knowledge concerning those developments and the sharing of benefits, with particular attention to the needs of developing countries;

(g) to safeguard and promote the interests of the present and future generations;

(h) to underline the importance of biodiversity and its conservation as a common concern of humankind.

Principles

Within the scope of this Declaration, in decisions or practices taken or carried out by those to whom it is addressed, the following principles are to be respected.

Article 3—Human dignity and human rights

1. Human dignity, human rights and fundamental freedoms are to be fully respected.
2. The interests and welfare of the individual should have priority over the sole interest of science or society.

Article 4—Benefit and harm

In applying and advancing scientific knowledge, medical practice and associated technologies, direct and indirect benefits to patients, research participants and other affected individuals should be maximized and any possible harm to such individuals should be minimized.

Article 5—Autonomy and individual responsibility

The autonomy of persons to make decisions, while taking responsibility for those decisions and respecting the autonomy of others, is to be respected. For persons who are not capable of exercising autonomy, special measures are to be taken to protect their rights and interests.

Article 6—Consent

1. Any preventive, diagnostic and therapeutic medical intervention is only to be carried out with the prior, free and informed consent of the person concerned, based on adequate information. The consent should, where appropriate, be express and may be withdrawn by the person concerned at any time and for any reason without disadvantage or prejudice.
2. Scientific research should only be carried out with the prior, free, express and informed consent of the person concerned. The information should be adequate, provided in a comprehensible form and should include modalities for withdrawal of consent. Consent may be withdrawn by the person concerned at any time and for any reason without any disadvantage or prejudice. Exceptions to this principle should be made only in accordance with ethical and legal standards adopted by States, consistent with the principles and provisions set out in this Declaration, in particular in Article 27, and international human rights law.
3. In appropriate cases of research carried out on a group of persons or a community, additional agreement of the legal representatives of the group or community concerned may be sought. In no case should a collective community agreement or the consent of a community leader or other authority substitute for an individual's informed consent.

Article 7—Persons without the capacity to consent

In accordance with domestic law, special protection is to be given to persons who do not have the capacity to consent:
   (a) authorization for research and medical practice should be obtained in accordance with the best interest of the person concerned and in accordance with domestic law. However, the person concerned should be involved to the greatest extent possible in the decision-making process of consent, as well as that of withdrawing consent;
   (b) research should only be carried out for his or her direct health benefit, subject to the authorization and the protective conditions prescribed by law, and if there is no research alternative of comparable

effectiveness with research participants able to consent. Research which does not have potential direct health benefit should only be undertaken by way of exception, with the utmost restraint, exposing the person only to a minimal risk and minimal burden and, if the research is expected to contribute to the health benefit of other persons in the same category, subject to the conditions prescribed by law and compatible with the protection of the individual's human rights. Refusal of such persons to take part in research should be respected.

Article 8—Respect for human vulnerability and personal integrity

In applying and advancing scientific knowledge, medical practice and associated technologies, human vulnerability should be taken into account. Individuals and groups of special vulnerability should be protected and the personal integrity of such individuals respected.

Article 9—Privacy and confidentiality

The privacy of the persons concerned and the confidentiality of their personal information should be respected. To the greatest extent possible, such information should not be used or disclosed for purposes other than those for which it was collected or consented to, consistent with international law, in particular international human rights law.

Article 10—Equality, justice and equity

The fundamental equality of all human beings in dignity and rights is to be respected so that they are treated justly and equitably.

Article 11—Non-discrimination and non-stigmatization

No individual or group should be discriminated against or stigmatized on any grounds, in violation of human dignity, human rights and fundamental freedoms.

Article 12—Respect for cultural diversity and pluralism

The importance of cultural diversity and pluralism should be given due regard. However, such considerations are not to be invoked to infringe upon human dignity, human rights and fundamental freedoms, nor upon the principles set out in this Declaration, nor to limit their scope.

Article 13—Solidarity and cooperation

Solidarity among human beings and international cooperation towards that end are to be encouraged.

Article 14—Social responsibility and health

1. The promotion of health and social development for their people is a central purpose of governments that all sectors of society share.
2. Taking into account that the enjoyment of the highest attainable standard of health is one of the fundamental rights of every human being without distinction of race, religion, political belief, economic or social condition, progress in science and technology should advance:
   (a) access to quality health care and essential medicines, especially for the health of women and children, because health is essential to life itself and must be considered to be a social and human good;
   (b) access to adequate nutrition and water;
   (c) improvement of living conditions and the environment;
   (d) elimination of the marginalization and the exclusion of persons on the basis of any grounds;
   (e) reduction of poverty and illiteracy.

Article 15—Sharing of benefits

1. Benefits resulting from any scientific research and its applications should be shared with society as a whole and within the international community, in particular with developing countries. In giving effect to this principle, benefits may take any of the following forms:
   (a) special and sustainable assistance to, and acknowledgement of, the persons and groups that have taken part in the research;
   (b) access to quality health care;
   (c) provision of new diagnostic and therapeutic modalities or products stemming from research;
   (d) support for health services;
   (e) access to scientific and technological knowledge;
   (f) capacity-building facilities for research purposes;
   (g) other forms of benefit consistent with the principles set out in this Declaration.
2. Benefits should not constitute improper inducements to participate in research.

Article 16—Protecting future generations

The impact of life sciences on future generations, including on their genetic constitution, should be given due regard.

Article 17—Protection of the environment, the biosphere and biodiversity

Due regard is to be given to the interconnection between human beings and other forms of life, to the importance of appropriate access and utilization of biological and genetic resources, to respect for traditional knowledge and to the role of human beings in the protection of the environment, the biosphere and biodiversity.

Application of the Principles
Article 18—Decision-making and addressing bioethical issues

1. Professionalism, honesty, integrity and transparency in decision-making should be promoted, in particular declarations of all conflicts of interest and appropriate sharing of knowledge. Every endeavour should be made to use the best available scientific knowledge and methodology in addressing and periodically reviewing bioethical issues.
2. Persons and professionals concerned and society as a whole should be engaged in dialogue on a regular basis.
3. Opportunities for informed pluralistic public debate, seeking the expression of all relevant opinions, should be promoted.

Article 19—Ethics committees

Independent, multidisciplinary and pluralist ethics committees should be established, promoted and supported at the appropriate level in order to:
  (a) assess the relevant ethical, legal, scientific and social issues related to research projects involving human beings;
  (b) provide advice on ethical problems in clinical settings;
  (c) assess scientific and technological developments, formulate recommendations and contribute to the preparation of guidelines on issues within the scope of this Declaration;
  (d) foster debate, education and public awareness of, and engagement in, bioethics.

Article 20—Risk assessment and management

Appropriate assessment and adequate management of risk related to medicine, life sciences and associated technologies should be promoted.

Article 21—Transnational practices

1. States, public and private institutions, and professionals associated with transnational activities should endeavour to ensure that any activity within the scope of this Declaration, undertaken, funded or otherwise pursued in whole or in part in different States, is consistent with the principles set out in this Declaration.
2. When research is undertaken or otherwise pursued in one or more States (the host State(s)) and funded by a source in another State, such research should be the object of an appropriate level of ethical review in the host State(s) and the State in which the funder is located. This review should be based on ethical and legal standards that are consistent with the principles set out in this Declaration.
3. Transnational health research should be responsive to the needs of host countries, and the importance of research contributing to the alleviation of urgent global health problems should be recognized.
4. When negotiating a research agreement, terms for collaboration and agreement on the benefits of research should be established with equal participation by those party to the negotiation.
5. States should take appropriate measures, both at the national and international levels, to combat bioterrorism and illicit traffic in organs, tissues, samples, genetic resources and genetic-related materials.

Promotion of the Declaration

Article 22—Role of States

1. States should take all appropriate measures, whether of a legislative, administrative or other character, to give effect to the principles set out in this Declaration in accordance with international human rights law. Such measures should be supported by action in the spheres of education, training and public information.
2. States should encourage the establishment of independent, multidisciplinary and pluralist ethics committees, as set out in Article 19.

Article 23—Bioethics education, training and information

1. In order to promote the principles set out in this Declaration and to achieve a better understanding of the ethical implications of scientific and technological developments, in particular for young people, States should endeavour to foster bioethics education and training at all levels

as well as to encourage information and knowledge dissemination pro-grammes about bioethics.

2. States should encourage the participation of international and regional intergovernmental organizations and international, regional and national non-governmental organizations in this endeavour.

Article 24—International cooperation

1. States should foster international dissemination of scientific information and encourage the free flow and sharing of scientific and technological knowledge.

2. Within the framework of international cooperation, States should pro-mote cultural and scientific cooperation and enter into bilateral and mul-tilateral agreements enabling developing countries to build up their capacity to participate in generating and sharing scientific knowledge, the related know-how and the benefits thereof.

3. States should respect and promote solidarity between and among States, as well as individuals, families, groups and communities, with special regard for those rendered vulnerable by disease or disability or other per-sonal, societal or environmental conditions and those with the most lim-ited resources.

Article 25—Follow-up action by UNESCO

1. UNESCO shall promote and disseminate the principles set out in this Declaration. In doing so, UNESCO should seek the help and assistance of the Intergovernmental Bioethics Committee (IGBC) and the Interna-tional Bioethics Committee (IBC).

2. UNESCO shall reaffirm its commitment to dealing with bioethics and to promoting collaboration between IGBC and IBC.

Final Provisions

Article 26—Interrelation and complementarity of the principles

This Declaration is to be understood as a whole and the principles are to be understood as complementary and interrelated. Each principle is to be considered in the context of the other principles, as appropriate and relevant in the circumstances.

Article 27—Limitations on the application of the principles

If the application of the principles of this Declaration is to be limited, it should be by law, including laws in the interests of public safety, for the investigation, detection and prosecution of criminal offences, for the protection of public health or for the protection of the rights and freedoms of others. Any such law needs to be consistent with international human rights law.

Article 28—Denial of acts contrary to human rights,
fundamental freedoms and human dignity

Nothing in this Declaration may be interpreted as implying for any State, group or person any claim to engage in any activity or to perform any act contrary to human rights, fundamental freedoms and human dignity.

NOTES

Preface and Acknowledgments

1. Jones, "Concept of Natural Theology in the Gifford Lectures"; Jones, *Earnest Enquirers after Truth*; Jaki, *Lord Gifford and His Lectures*; Witham, *Measure of God*.
2. Gifford, "Trust, Disposition and Settlement," 74.
3. Ibid., 72.

Introduction: The Hippocratic Problem

1. AMA, CEJA, *Code of Medical Ethics* (2010), xiii.
2. See "Hippocratic Oath," under "A-Z of Common Queries and Useful Websites," *British Medical Association*, www.bma.org.uk/patients_public/AZusefulsites.jsp#Hippo cratic%20Oath, accessed January 5, 2012.
3. Adams, "Expert: Conrad Murray Violated Hippocratic Oath When Treating Michael Jackson," *Crime Examiner*, www.examiner.com/crime-in-national/expert-con rad-murray-violated-hippocratic-oath-when-treating-michael-jackson, accessed January 5, 2012.
4. "Jackson Family Statement from Brain Panish," *JanetJackson.com*, December 1, 2011. www.janetjackson.com/story/news/jackson-family-statement-from-brian-panish, accessed January 5, 2012.
5. Pat Patrick, "Judge Pastor Sentenced Conrad Murray to Four Years Imprisonment," *Chicago Community Life Examiner*, November 29, 2011, www.examiner.com/com munity-life-in-chicago/judge-pastor-sentenced-conrad-murray-to-four-years-imprisonment, accessed January 5, 2012.
6. Miles, *Hippocratic Oath and the Ethics of Medicine*, vii.
7. Jonsen, Siegler, and Winslade, *Clinical Ethics*, 10, 174.
8. Frankel, Lorry R., Amnon Goldworth, Mary V. Rorty, and William A. Silverman, eds. *Ethical Dilemmas in Pediatrics: Cases and Commentaries*. New York: Cambridge University Press, 2005, 1.
9. AMA, *Code of Medical Ethics* (1848), 15–16.
10. Ibid., 16.

Chapter 1: The Hippocratic Oath and the Ethic of Hippocratism

1. Jones, *Doctor's Oath*, 2.
2. Edelstein, "Hippocratic Oath," 55.
3. Ibid. I will generally use the Edelstein translation of the Oath unless otherwise noted. For other translations, see Jones, *Doctor's Oath*; and von Staden, "'In a Pure and Holy Way.'" The translations are, of course, the work of the translators, so variations in tone, nuance, and meaning are inevitable. Even the Greek versions available represent a wide range of manuscripts, the earliest and most reliable of which date from no earlier than the tenth century of the common era, some 1,500 years after the supposed original writing. For a good summary of the problems and variations in the manuscript texts, see Jones, *Doctor's Oath*. Jones hints at Pythagorean connections for the Oath prior to the work of Edelstein (45).
4. Matthai, "*Tractatus de philosophia medici sive*," 108.
5. Carrick, *Medical Ethics in Antiquity*, 162–63; Kudlien, "Medical Ethics and Popular Ethics," 104, 107ff; von Staden, "'In a Pure and Holy Way'"; and Prioreschi, "Hippocratic Oath." Kudlien refers to the "pan-pythagorizing trend" of eighteenth-century medicine.
6. Edelstein, "Hippocratic Oath," 6.
7. Ibid.
8. Meyer, "Truth and the Physician."
9. The claim here is not that benefit must be assessed based on the personal preferences of the patient. That is one, but only one, alternative. The good for the patient may rest on some objective teleology such as seen in Christian natural law theory. Thus, Allen Verhey misunderstands the nature of the problem. See Verhey, "The Doctor's Oath," 155–56, where he accuses me of reducing patient benefit to private personal preferences external to the practice of medicine. He is correct that the good for the patient must be external to the practice of medicine but wrong in assuming that the external standard for the good for the patient must reduce to personal preferences. The external source may be a more objective theory of the good such as that reflected in traditional Christian teleological natural law theory. What is problematic in the Hippocratic paternalistic formulation is that the good is necessarily known best by the physician's judgment. In Christian natural law theory, for example, it is far more plausible that theological experts in natural law theory would be considered the authoritative standard than some individual medical practitioner. Other objective theories of the good might turn to other external standards for assessing the patient's good. For further discussion of this problem, see Veatch, "Impossibility of a Morality Internal to Medicine."
10. I first developed this formulation of these three characteristics of the Hippocratic Oath in Veatch, "The Hippocratic Ethic: Consequentialism, Individualism and Paternalism."
11. Edelstein, "Hippocratic Oath," 6.
12. An alternative interpretation of the Hippocratic text reads this section as prohibiting physician participation in homicide, that is, garden-variety murder through the use

of poison, a subject about which the physician can be understood to be an expert. Edelstein rejects this interpretation (9ff), but others have found it more plausible, basing their reading on the fact that, in ancient Greek culture, physicians were known to have collaborated in homicide. *See* Kudlien, "Medical Ethics and Popular Ethics," 101 and n47. If this reading were correct, there would be even more reason to argue that the Hippocratic Oath is not relevant to twenty-first century society. Surely a code of ethics is not needed for physicians and others to understand that it is immoral for physicians to conspire in murder.

13. Edelstein, "Hippocratic Oath," 17n45, 62; Carrick, *Medical Ethics in Antiquity*, 66, 159; and Verhey, "The Doctor's Oath," 157, 170.

14. Kevorkian, *Prescription Medicide*.

15. *Michigan v. Kevorkian*, No. 221758, (Oakland Cir. Ct. Mar. 16, 1999); and *People v. Kevorkian*, 248 Mich. App. 373, 639 N.W.2d 291 (Ct. App. 2001).

16. Review procedures of termination of life on request and assisted suicide and amendment to the Penal Code and the Burial and Cremation Act. Senate, session 2000–2001, 26 691, no. 137 (Netherlands Euthanasia Law). More recently, Belgium has adopted a similar policy. "Oregon Death with Dignity Act (Ballot Measure 16)." *Trends in Health Care, Law and Ethics* 9, no. 4 (1994): 29–32. In 2008 the state of Washington also accepted physician-assisted suicide (Revised Code of Washington, Chapter 70.245 "The Washington Death with Dignity Act," enacted November 4, 2008 (http://apps.leg.wa.gov/RCW/default.aspx?cite=70.245, accessed November 8, 2010), and in 2009 a court in Montana determined that such assistance was not contrary to Montana law (*Baxter et al. v. Montana* in the Supreme Court of the State of Montana 2009 Mt 449, December 31, 2009).

17. Edelstein, "Hippocratic Oath," 18ff.

18. Kudlien, "Medical Ethics and Popular Ethics," 109.

19. In particular, von Staden, "'In a Pure and Holy Way.'"

20. Edelstein, "Hippocratic Oath," 32.

21. Verhey, "Doctor's Oath," 144–45. Verhey's rationalization of the prohibition on surgery as an injunction not to go beyond one's competence fails to explain why surgery should be deemed beyond any Hippocratic physician's competence. The Oath provides a clear differentiation between Hippocratic physicians, who are not to practice surgery, and others who are engaged in that work, leaving open the question of why Hippocratic physicians would never be so engaged.

22. In von Staden's extended analysis of the significance of the virtue of purity, he struggles with the meaning for the Hippocratic physician. He rejects the rigorist imperative to remain at all times free from contaminating pollution (such as from blood) on the grounds that it is impossible for any human, let alone a physician, to lead a "perfectly pure" life. On the other hand, he rejects the alternative that sees the Hippocratic physician enjoined to lead periods of religious purity alongside periods of "temporary pollution" followed by repurification." von Staden, "'In a Pure and Holy Way,'" 425.

23. Edelstein, "Hippocratic Oath," 6.

24. "General Medical Council," 79–80.

25. *Tarasoff v. Regents of the University of California Supreme Court of California*, 1974 13 Cal. 3d 177.

26. AMA, CEJA, *Code of Medical Ethics* (2006).

27. von Staden, "'In a Pure and Holy Way,'" 420.

28. AMA, CEJA, *Code of Medical Ethics* (2008), 149.

29. Edelstein, "Hippocratic Oath, 6.

30. See von Staden, "'In a Pure and Holy Way,'" 408–10.

31. Jones, *Doctor's Oath*, 45–46, suggests that other Hippocratic writings including the *Precepts, Decorum*, and the *Law* also have qualities resembling addresses to secret societies. *Law* actually ends with an injunction that the profane (that is, ordinary people) may not be shown the things presented.

32. Kudlien, "Medical Ethics and Popular Ethics," 110, refers to "mysterious cults." He notes that the professional guild was, at least originally, religious and therefore esoteric.

33. Roth, "Medicine's Ethical Responsibilities," 1957.

34. Brock, "Euthanasia," 662.

35. That is the central thesis of my recent book where the claim is argued at length. Veatch, *Patient, Heal Thyself.*

36. Veatch, "Generalization of Expertise."

Chapter 2: The Hippocratic Tradition

1. Plato, *Protagorus*, 331b–c; and *Phaedrus*, 170b–d. See also Carrick, *Medical Ethics in Antiquity*, 76.

2. Kudlien, "Medical Ethics and Popular Ethics."

3. Jones, *Doctor's Oath*, 39.

4. Ibid., 44.

5. Galvao-Sobrinho, "Hippocratic Ideals."

6. Garzya, "Science et conscience."

7. Jouanna, "La lecture de l'éthiquee Hippocratique."

8. Veatch and Mason, "Hippocratic vs. Judeo-Christian Medical Ethics."

9. Jerome, "Letter LII," 95. Since Jerome refers to matters of gait, dress, and manners that are not addressed in existing copies of the Oath, scholars have suggested either that Jerome had access to a variant text or that he presented only a rough summary of the content of the Oath. See Jones, *Doctor's Oath*, 41–42.

10. Gregory of Nazianzus, "Oration VII," 233.

11. Galvao-Sobrinho, "Hippocratic Ideals," 443–44.

12. Ibid., 444.

13. Cited in ibid.

14. Ibid., 445.

15. Ibid., 451.

16. A similar pattern is found by Galvao-Sobrinho when he examines the Visigothic Code of Germanic law. None of these laws seem informed by the Hippocratic Oath. For example, physician cooperation in suicide as a general practice was not addressed. Helping men of rank commit suicide was penalized only because their death was seen as diminishing public justice. Similarly, the Germanic law did not forbid surgery, and, while the law spelled out fees apprentices should pay their teachers, no provision was made for teaching of the master's sons, as was provided in the Oath. See ibid., 454–55.

17. Jones, *Doctor's Oath*, 23, 25. All references to this Christian form of the Oath are taken from Jones.

18. MacKinney, "Medical Ethics and Etiquette," 12, provides translation of a Chartes manuscript addressing what sort of a person a physician ought to be. It states the physician should "be mindful of the Hippocratic Oath." The text incorporates other moral instruction, however, that is alien to the Oath. It says the physician "should take care of rich and poor, slave and free, equally for among all such people medicines are needed." Also, MacKinney provides text of two additional manuscripts of this period that make explicit reference to physicians taking the Hippocratic Oath (ibid., 15–16). These texts also contain non-Hippocratic themes—the practice of surgery, for example.

19. At least that is the earliest manuscript to which MacKinney makes reference. Ibid., 19n29.

20. Jones, *Doctor's Oath*.

21. Ibid., 4.

22. Ibid., 52, 55.

23. English translation in ibid., 23.

24. Jones is puzzled by the omission of the secrecy clause, which he takes as encouraging "the formation of an inner ring of physicians from which outsiders were carefully excluded." He considers that the Christian version merely derived from a version of the pagan oath that omitted the "inner circle" as well as an intentional effort of the Christian compiler to avoid encouraging a trade union. While he considers the second explanation more likely, he fails to see the pagan text as reflecting a Greek mystery cult, which would, of course, be anathema to Christians.

25. Jones, *Doctor's Oath*, 23.

26. Ibid., 25. The fact that this concluding section of the Oath is a problem for Christians is suggested by the variation in the surviving redactions. Bononiensis omits some of the words, and both Urbinas and Ambrosianus have textual problems as well. See ibid., 25n1–3.

27. MacKinney, "Medical Ethics and Etiquette," 2.

28. Ibid., 25.

29. Ibid.

30. Text translated in ibid., 26.

31. The discussion of Arabic texts and French sources here is heavily dependent on the research assistance of Yashar Saghai, for which I am grateful.

32. Jacquart, "Le sens donné par Constantin," 78.

33. Ibid.
34. Strohmaier, "Hunayn Ibn Ishaq et le Serment d'Hippocrate."
35. Larijani and Zahedi, "Introductory on Medical Ethics."
36. Levey. *Medical Ethics of Medieval Islam.*
37. Habbi, "Le role de Hunayn," 297.
38. Habbi, "L'eredita Ippocratica."
39. Rosner, *Medical Legacy of Moses Maimonides*; and Rosner, "Life of Moses Maimonides."
40. Larkey, "Hippocratic Oath in Elizabethan England," 201.
41. Ibid.
42. Schleiner, *Medical Ethics in the Renaissance.*
43. Ibid.
44. Ibid., 77.
45. Rodrigo de Castro, *Medicus Politicus*, Hamburg, 1614, 86, cited in Schleiner, 71.
46. Schleiner, *Medical Ethics in the Renaissance*, 108.
47. Ibid.
48. Maclean, *Renaissance Notion of Woman*, 29.
49. Schleiner, *Medical Ethics in the Renaissance*, 75; Smith, *Hippocratic Tradition*, 216–17; Temkin, *Hippocrates in a World of Pagans and Christians*, 57–75.
50. Schleiner, *Medical Ethics in the Renaissance*, viii, 17, 25.
51. Ibid.
52. Pomis, David de, *De medico Hebraeo enarratio apologetica.* Venice, 1588, 12, cited in Schleiner, *Medical Ethics in the Renaissance*, 69.
53. Ibid., 33–35, from which this account is adapted. The first volume is titled *Record University of Edinburgh Laureations and Degrees 1585 to 1896*, Registry Office, University of Edinburgh. I'm grateful to the staff of the special collections of the library and the Registry Office for helpful assistance in gaining access to these volumes.
54. Dalzel, *History of the University of Edinburgh*, 100.
55. The full text appears in the first volume of the Laureation book above Cockburn's name. It is reprinted in the 1846 compendium of all medical school graduates up to that time. See "Nomina Eorum, qui gradum Medicinae Doctoris in Academia Jacobi Sexti Scotorum Regis, quae Edinburgi est, Adepti Sunt. Edinburgh: Exciebant Neill et Soch, 1846" [Edinburgh medical graduates, 1705–1845].
56. The full text (taken from Veatch, *Disrupted Dislogue*, 34) reads:

> Whereas the distinction of a degree in Medicine is now to be conferred upon me, I solemnly promise before God, the Searcher of hearts, that I will to my latest breath abide steadfast in all due loyalty to the University of Edinburgh. Further, that I will practise the art of Medicine with care, with purity of conduct and with uprightness, and, so far as in me lies, will faithfully attend to everything conducive to the welfare of the sick. Lastly, that, whatever things seen or heard in the course of medical practice which ought not to be spoken of, I will not, save for right reason, divulge. This I promise, as I hope for the gracious blessing of Heaven.

57. Gregory, *Lectures on the Duties and Qualifications of a Physician.*

58. The documentation of this claim is provided in Veatch, *Disrupted Dialogue,* 15–16.

59. For example, [Percival], *Philosophical, Medical, and Experimental Essays;* Percival, *Moral and Literary Dissertations;* and Percival, *Works, Literary, Moral, and Philosophical.*

60. See Veatch, *Disrupted Dialogue,* 56–70.

61. For the documentation, see ibid., 69–70.

62. For detailed documentation, see ibid., 85–95.

63. [Commission for Visiting the Universities and Colleges in Scotland], *Evidence, Oral and Documentary.*

64. Warren, Hayward, and Fleet, "Boston Medical Police," 41–46.

65. See Veatch, *Disrupted Dialogue,* 103–7.

66. Warren, Hayward, and Fleet, "Boston Medical Police," 41.

67. Medical Society of the State of New York, *System of Medical Ethics.*

68. Medico–Chirurgical Society of Baltimore, *System of Medical Ethics;* and Medical Association of the District of Columbia, *Regulations and System of Ethics.*

69. Walsh, *History of the Medical Society,* 148.

70. See Veatch, *Disrupted Dialogue,* 110–14.

71. Kappa Lambda, "Formula to Be Observed."

72. See the text of this portion of the initiation ceremony in Veatch, *Disrupted Dialogue,* 111.

73. Kappa Lambda, "Formula to Be Observed."

74. Kappa Lambda, *Constitution and By-Laws.*

75. Sandys, *History of Classical Scholarship,* 2:479.

76. Ibid., 3:252.

77. Ibid., iii–iv.

78. Adams, *Genuine Works of Hippocrates,* v.

79. Baker et al., *American Medical Ethics Revolution;* Baker, "Historical Context of the AMA's 1847 *Code of Ethics*"; McCrae, "Hays, Isaac," in *Dictionary of American Biography,* ed. Allen Johnson and Dumas Malone, 462–63; and Bell, "Introduction to the Code of Medical Ethics."

80. AMA, *Code of Medical Ethics* (1848).

81. Ibid., 13.

82. Ibid., 14–15.

83. Ibid., 15–16.

84. Ibid., 22.

85. McLean, *First Do No Harm,* 2006; Donaldson, *Do No Harm;* and Burgio and Lantos, eds., *Primum non nocere Today.*

86. Sandulescu, *"Primum non nocere"*; Jonsen, "Do No Harm"; and Veatch, *Theory of Medical Ethics,* 161.

87. Smith, "Origin and Uses of *Primum non nocere,*" 372, citing T. Inman, *Foundation for a New Theory and Practice of Medicine.*

88. Veatch, *Patient, Heal Thyself.*

89. AMA, CEJA, *Code of Medical Ethics* (2008), xi.

90. AMA, "Principles of Medical Ethics."

91. Todd, "Report of the Ad Hoc Committee."

92. AMA, *Current Opinion of the Judicial Council*, ix.

93. *Tarasoff v. Regents of the University of California*, Supreme Court of California, 1974 13 Cal. 3d 177 (1974).

94. Todd, "Report of the Ad Hoc Committee," 1.

95. Burns, "Reciprocity in the Development," 304.

96. "General Medical Council," 79–80.

97. "Central Ethical Committee," *British Medical Journal Supplement* (May 1, 1971), 30.

98. Lifton, *Nazi Doctors*; Annas and Grodin, eds. *Nazi Doctors and the Nuremberg Code*; Rozenberg, ed. *Bioethical and Ethical Issues*; and Caplan, "Ethics of Evil."

99. Veatch, "Nazis and Hippocratists."

100. World Medical Association, "Declaration of Geneva."

101. "Nuremberg Code, 1947," in *Encyclopedia of Bioethics*, rev. ed., vol. 5, ed. Warren T. Reich (New York: Free Press, 1995), 2763–64.

102. Ibid., 2764.

103. Ibid., 2763.

Chapter 3: The Cacophony of Codes

1. "Dean Gotto Unveils Revised Hippocratic Oath for New Generation of Weill Cornell Graduates," *Weill Cornell Medical College*, www.med.cornell.edu/deans/2005/07_01_05/article_4-7_1.shtml, accessed November 11, 2010.

2. "Hippocratic Oath" (2005), *Weill Cornell Medical College*, www.med.cornell.edu/deans/pdf/hippocratic_oath.pdf, accessed November 11, 2010.

3. The replacement of "purity" with "integrity" is suggestive. Some modern virtue theorists working in medical ethics have suggested that purity today may be taken in the sense of "lack of contamination," in particular, lack of contaminating influences in the physician's dedication to single-minded devotion to healing, free from concern about fame or income. This is a line worthy of pursuit if one is developing a virtue theory for medicine. I think it is probable that this was not the meaning of the original Hippocratic language.

4. "A Revised Hippocratic Oath," *Weill Cornell Medical College*, www.med.cornell.edu/publichealth/divisions/medical_ethics/revised_hippocratic.html, accessed November 11, 2010.

5. "Hippocratic Oath" (2005), *Weill Cornell Medical College*.

6. Veatch and Macpherson, "Medical School Oath-Taking."

7. We asked them for their student ID number so we could match their responses to a planned repeat of the question after the students had completed their ethics courses.

We promised them we would not attempt to use their ID number to identify them or for any purpose other than matching their two responses.

Chapter 4: The Limits of Professionally Generated Ethics

1. Pellegrino, "Goals and Ends of Medicine"; Pellegrino, "Internal Morality of Clinical Medicine"; Brody and Miller, "Internal Morality of Medicine"; and Miller and Brody, "Professional Integrity and Physician-assisted Death."

2. See Pellegrino, "Internal Morality of Clinical Medicine," 564–65. For an example of someone relying on the internal morality thesis but is not as careful to acknowledge that laypeople can also arrive at this knowledge, see Paul, "Internal and External Morality of Medicine."

3. Russo, "Ethical Use of Pharmacologic Fatigue Countermeasures."

4. Gordon, Gerjuoy, and Anderson, eds., *Life-Extending Technologies*.

5. Walford, *Maximum Life Span*; and Woodhead, Blackett, and Hollaender, *Molecular Biology of Aging*; Hayflick, "Theories of Biological Aging"; Shock, "Physiological Basis of Aging."

6. Mehlman, *Wondergenes*; Zylinska, "Playing God, Playing Adam"; and Savulescu and Bostrom, *Human Enhancement*.

7. Mehlman, *Wondergenes*; Zylinska, "Playing God, Playing Adam"; and Savulescu and Bostrom, eds., *Human Enhancement*.

8. Meilaender, "On Removing Food and Water."

9. Callahan, "On Feeding the Dying."

10. AMA, *Current Opinions of the Council on Ethical and Judicial Affairs*, sec. 2.20, 13.

11. Ibid., sec. 2.21, 13.

12. Sulmasy, "Terri Schiavo." Note, however, that recent Vatican writing on the subject of withholding of nutrition and hydration has become more critical of treating these as extraordinary means. See Hamel and Walter, eds. *Artificial Nutrition and Hydration*; and Tollefsen, ed., *Artificial Nutrition and Hydration*. The latter includes Pope John Paul II's 2004 statement "Care for Patients in a 'Permanent' Vegetative State."

13. AMA, CEJA, *Code of Medical Ethics* (1994), sec. 2.20, 37.

14. AMA, CEJA, "Physician Participation in Capital Punishment."

15. "WMA Resolution on Physician Participation in Capital Punishment," adopted in 1981 and reaffirmed as amended in 2008. *World Medical Association*, www.wma.net/en/30publications/10policies/c1/index.html, accessed November 23, 2010; and "Recommendations from *The Medical Profession and Human Rights: Handbook for a Changing Agenda*," *British Medical Association*, September 7, 2006, www.bma.org.uk/ethics/human_rights/MedProfhumanRightsRecommendations.jsp#Capitalandcorporalpunishment, accessed November 23, 2010. See resolutions 24–29.

16. AMA, CEJA, *Code of Medical Ethics* (2008), 20–21.

17. Ibid., 21.

18. Ibid.

19. "Anesthesiologists and Capital Punishment," *American Board of Anesthesiology*, www.theaba.org/Home/notices#punishment, accessed November 23, 2010.

20. Rockoff, Mark A., "Commentary: Anesthesiologists and Capital Punishment," April 2, 2010. *American Board of Anesthesiologists*. Available at http://www.theaba.org/pdf/CapitalPunishmentCommentary.pdf, accessed May 8, 2012.

21. See United States Conference of Catholic Bishops, "Catholic Campaign."

22. Bernardin, *Seamless Garment*.

23. "On Capital Punishment, June 2000," *SBC Resolutions*, www.sbc.net/resolutions/amResolution.asp?ID = 299, accessed November 22, 2010.

24. See "Death Penalty: Policies of Various Religious Groups," *ReligiousTolerance.org*, www.religioustolerance.org/execut7.htm, accessed November 22, 2010.

25. See "Capital Punishment: The Ultimate Denial of Civil Liberties," *American Civil Liberties Union*, www.aclu.org/capital-punishment, accessed November 22, 2010.

26. "Republican Party Platform on Crime," *On the Issues*, www.ontheissues.org/celeb/Republican_Party_Crime.htm, accessed November 22, 2010.

27. AMA, CEJA, *Code of Medical Ethics* (2008), 81.

Chapter 5: Religious Medical Ethics

1. United States Conference of Catholic Bishops. *Ethical and Religious Directives*; "Declaration on Euthanasia," Vatican website, www.vatican.va/roman_curia/congregations/cfaith/documents/rc_con_cfaith_doc_19800505_euthanasia_en.html; *"Humanae Vitae,"* Vatican website, www.vatican.va/holy_father/paul_vi/encyclicals/documents/hf_ep-vi_enc_25071968_humanae-vitae_en.html; and "Declaration on the Production and the Scientific and Therapeutic Use of Human Embryonic Stem Cells," Vatican website, www.vatican.va/roman_curia/pontifical_academies/acdlife/documents/rc_pa_acdlife_doc_20000824_cellule-staminali_en.html.

2. Kappa Lambda, "Formula to Be Observed."

3. For further information and the text of their non-Hippocratic Oath, see Veatch, *Disrupted Dialogue*, 110–13. The organization had chapters in Philadelphia, New York, Baltimore, Washington, and Lexington.

4. Barth, *Knowledge of God.*

5. Gifford, "Trust, Disposition and Settlement, 74.

6. Barth, *Knowledge of God*, ix.

7. Ibid., 5.

8. Ibid., ix.

9. Ibid., 26.

10. Ibid., 103.

11. Ibid.

12. Ibid., 104.

13. I rely on the 1981 one-volume English translation, edited by Dietrich Braun and translated by Geoffrey W. Bromiley.

14. Ibid., 13.

15. Ibid., 12.

16. Ibid.

17. Ibid., 19.

18. Ibid., 20.

19. Ibid.

20. Barth, *Church Dogmatics*. I am grateful to Stephen E. Lammers and Allen Verhey, two contemporary theologically oriented bioethicists, for their extensive anthology of theological writing in bioethics that helps point the way toward Barth's sparse words relevant to bioethics in his massive writings. *See* Lammers and Verhey, eds, *On Moral Medicine*.

21. Barth, *Church Dogmatics*, III/4, 324.

22. Ibid., 324.

23. Ibid., 325.

24. Ibid., 339.

25. Ibid., 419.

26. Ibid., 417.

27. Ibid., 418.

28. Ibid., 270.

29. Lambeth Conference, *Encyclical Letter*.

30. Barth, *Church Dogmatics*, III/4, 271.

31. Ibid., 356.

32. Ibid., 361.

33. Ibid. I would argue that Barth is wrong even in the psychological and physical spheres of well-being. I have claimed elsewhere that even organic well-being requires a complex set of value judgments, for example, in assigning relative weights to preserving life, curing disease, relieving suffering, and preserving health. These are all legitimate organic goods, but they often compete, and when they do, there is no definitive, objective basis for choosing one particular balance of the competing medical goods. Moreover, even if one could determine the proper mix of medical goods, no rational person wishes to be maximally healthy since achieving that amount of medical good would require the sacrifice of other goods in various nonmedical spheres. One cannot spend all her time pursuing health because doing so would jeopardize important pursuits in the spiritual, social, familial, aesthetic, and other spheres of life that deserve their fair share of a person's time and resources. See Veatch, *Patient, Heal Thyself*.

34. Barth, *Church Dogmatics*, III/4, 357, and on a number of occasions in the following pages.

35. Ibid., 357.

36. Ibid., 361.

37. Hauerwas, *With the Grain of the Universe*.

38. As Hauerwas acknowledges (18), another Gifford lecturer (and a Hauerwas mentor), Alasdair MacIntyre, also provides something of a challenge to Lord Gifford's mandate but does so by challenging the assumption apparently made by Lord Gifford that

natural theology must rely on an account of rationality that is present in the natural sciences. That is not the same as rejecting natural theology whole cloth. Hauerwas, himself, probably influenced by MacIntyre, sometimes also talks as if he is reconstructing natural theology rather than destroying it. See MacIntyre, *Three Rival Versions of Moral Enquiry*. Hauerwas acknowledges that his project is a more radical assault on the apparent intention Lord Gifford states in his trust because MacIntyre at least reflects a "profound commitment to philosophy as a master science" (Hauerwas, *With the Grain of the Universe*, 20) while Hauerwas works as a theologian, and an explicitly Barthian one at that.

39. Hauerwas, *With the Grain of the Universe*, 20.

40. Ibid., 20. The counterintuitive thesis is repeated almost verbatim on page 39 where Hauerwas says, "The great natural theologian of the Gifford Lectures is Karl Barth, for Barth, in contrast to James and Niebuhr, provides a robust theological description of existence." For Hauerwas "describing existence" becomes what is "natural" about natural theology even if that description is based solely on revealed, not natural, knowledge.

41. Hauerwas, *Suffering Presence*, 71.

42. Ibid., 72.

43. Ibid., 73.

44. Ibid., 36.

45. Ibid., 142.

46. Ibid., 143.

47. Harrell, *Oral Roberts*; and Roberts, *Expect a Miracle*.

48. See Baker and Ehlke, eds. *Natural Law*.

49. Oken, "What to Tell Cancer Patients."

50. Meyer, "Truth and the Physician."

51. Rosner, "Organ Transplantation in Jewish Law"; and Tendler, "Cessation of Brain Function."

52. Engelhardt, *Foundations of Bioethics*, 39.

53. Ibid., 69–72. Cf. Engelhardt, *Foundations of Bioethics*, 2nd ed., 103–31.

54. Engelhardt, *Foundations of Christian Bioethics*.

55. Ibid., 14–16.

56. Ibid., 157–59.

57. Ibid., 168.

58. Ibid., 168–72, especially n31.

59. Ibid., 169.

60. Ibid., 171.

61. Aquinas, *Summa theologica*, I-II, Q. 94.

62. Porter, *Natural and Divine Law*; Porter, *Nature as Reason*; and Porter, *Ministers of the Law*.

63. Porter, *Nature as Reason*, 5.

64. United States Conference of Catholic Bishops, *Ethical and Religious Directives*; McCormick, *Health and Medicine in the Catholic Tradition*; McFadden, *Medical Ethics*;

Kelly, *Medico-Moral Problems*; Healy, *Medical Ethics*; Haring, *Medical Ethics*; and O'Rourke and Boyle, *Medical Ethics*.

65. Sacred Congregation for the Doctrine of the Faith, *Declaration on Euthanasia*.

66. Haring, *Medical Ethics*, 131–36.

67. There, of course, have been exceptions. In the middle ages there were periods when priests served as physicians. On the other hand, in other periods priests were prohibited from practicing medicine so virtually all the experts in medical morality were not medical professionals. In contemporary times there are occasional members of religious orders who are also physicians. Daniel Sulmasy, OFM, MD, PhD, is a particularly vivid example. There are also serious Catholic laymen who are physicians who have been schooled very thoroughly in Catholic medical morality. Edmund Pellegrino, MD, the former president of Catholic University of America, my predecessor as director of the Kennedy Institute of Ethics, and recently chair of the President's Council on Bioethics, is notoriously humble when it comes to admitting expertise in Catholic moral theology, but, in fact, he is as knowledgeable as (or more knowledgeable than) many Catholic theologians and priests.

68. Berman, *Faith and Order*.

69. Ibid., 40.

70. Ibid., 41.

71. Vandrunen, "Context of Natural Law."

72. Methodism, of course, also had a huge impact on medical practice of the eighteenth century as well as later years. John Wesley, Methodism's founder, wrote what was apparently the best-selling medical book of the eighteenth century, a handbook for parishioners to take care of their own health. Wesley, *Primitive Physick*. Just as important, Methodism placed a strong emphasis on the virtues and healthful habits. The twentieth-century physician and social commentator called Wesley "one of the formative [health] influences on middle-class England." Morison, "Rights and Responsibilities," 3.

73. *The Book of Discipline of the United Methodist Church—2004*, 77; Thorsen, *Wesleyan Quadrilateral*; and Gunter, Jones, Campbell, Miles, and Maddox, *Wesley and the Quadrilateral*.

74. This notion of embedding a second-level ethic for professional conduct in a more general normative theory of ethics governing all human societal interaction was developed at some length in my early book, *A Theory of Medical Ethics*. In that work I proposed a "triple-contract" basis for medical ethics: a first-level general social contract for human morality; a second-level contract between medical professionals and laypeople to articulate the moral norms for conduct of the members of a profession (as well as the norms for conduct of laypeople when interacting with professionals) bounded by the more general, first-level moral norms; and a third-level contract between the individual patient and professional establishing the limits of behavior within the individual doctor–patient relation bounded by the two higher level contracts. See Veatch, *A Theory of Medical Ethics*, 108–38.

Chapter 6: Secular Ethics and Professional Ethics

1. Meyer, "Truth and the Physician." See also Oken, "What to Tell Cancer Patients." Cf. Cabot, "Use of Truth and Falsehood in Medicine."

2. Kant, "On the Supposed Right to Tell Lies."

3. Fletcher, *Morals and Medicine*, 34–64.

4. AMA, *Current Opinion of the Judicial Council.*

5. Rawls, *Theory of Justice.*

6. Daniels, *Just Health Care*; Green, "Health Care and Justice"; Veatch, *Foundations of Justice*; DeGrazia, "Grounding a Right to Health Care"; and Daniels and Sabin, *Setting Limits Fairly.*

7. Hutcheson, *Illustrations on the Moral Sense.*

8. Smith, *Theory of Moral Sentiments.*

9. Freedman, "Equipoise and the Ethics of Clinical Research"; and Weijer, "Clinical Equipoise"; Cf. Karlawish and Lantos, "Community Equipoise"; Gifford, "Community-Equipoise"; Ashcroft, "Equipoise, Knowledge and Ethics"; Miller and Brody, "Critique of Clinical Equipoise"; Veatch, "Indifference of Subjects"; and Veatch, "Irrelevance of Equipoise."

10. Novack, Detering, Arnold, Ladinsky, and Pezzullo, "Physician's Attitudes toward Using Deception," 2981.

11. Gregory, *Lectures on the Duties*. See also Veatch, *Disrupted Dialogue*, 15–16, for an account of Gregory's lack of interest in the Hippocratic ethic.

12. Perry, *Thought and Character of William James.*

13. James, *Essays in Radical Empiricism.*

14. Perry, *Realms of Value*, 90.

15. See Brandt, *Ethical Theory*, 169–72.

16. Perry, *Realms of Value*, 135.

17. Firth, "Ethical Absolutism."

18. Pellegrino and Thomasma, *For the Patient's Good*, 103, 105, 118, 154–55; and Cassell, *Healer's Art*, 44–45, 146, 163.

19. Lief and Fox, "Training for 'Detached Concern,'" 12–35.

20. For more developed analysis of this problem, see Veatch, *Value-Freedom in Science and Technology*, as well as Veatch and Stempsey, "Incommensurability."

21. Clouser, "Common Morality"; Gert, Culver, and Clouser, *Bioethics* (1997); Gert, Culver, and Clouser, "Common Morality versus Specified Principlism"; Gert, *Common Morality*; Gert, Culver, and Clouser, *Bioethics* (2006), 22–36.

22. Gert, Culver, and Clouser, *Bioethics* (1997), 16.

23. Ibid.

24. Ibid., 17.

25. Ibid., 18.

26. Beauchamp and Childress, *Principles of Biomedical Ethics*, 4th ed., 5–6, 37, 100–109; Beauchamp and Childress, *Principles of Biomedical Ethics*, 5th ed., 2–5, 401–8; Beauchamp, "Defense of the Common Morality"; Veatch, "Is There a Common Morality?";

DeGrazia, "Common Morality, Coherence, and the Principles of Biomedical Ethics"; Veatch, "Common Morality and Human Finitude," 37–50; Lindsay, "Slaves, Embryos, and Nonhuman Animals"; Veatch, "Benevolent Lies."

27. Beauchamp and Childress, *Principles of Biomedical Ethics*, 5th ed., 3.

28. Turner, "Zones of Consensus"; Turner, "Bioethics in a Multicultural World"; and Engelhardt, *Bioethics and Secular Humanism*.

29. National Research Act of 1974, Pub. L. No. 93–348, Title II–Protection of Human Subjects of Biomedical and Behavioral Research.

30. US Public Health Service, "Final Report of the Tuskegee Syphilis Study;" and Jones, *Bad Blood*.

31. Other trials are reviewed in Beecher, "Ethics and Clinical Research"; and Veatch, "Human Experimentation." The hearing proceedings are found in *Quality of Health Care—Human Experimentation, 1973: Hearings Before the Subcommittee on Health of the Committee on Labor and Public Welfare United States Senate*, 93rd Cong., 1st sess. on S. 974, S. 878, S.J. Res. 71: Part 1, February 21 and 22, 1973; Part 2, February 23 and March 6, 1973; Part 3, March 7 and 8, 1973; and Part 4, April 30, June 28, 29, and July 10, 1973.

32. Ibid., Part 1, February 21 and 22, 1973.

33. Ibid. (Statement of Robert Veatch, PhD, Hastings Institute, Hastings-on-Hudson, NY), 265–75.

34. Childress, Meslin, and Shapiro, eds. *Belmont Revisited*.

Chapter 7: Fallibilism and the Convergence Hypothesis

1. Veatch and Stempsey, "Incommensurability." For a fuller account of my views on the inevitability of systems of belief and value in even completely accurate accounts of reality see Veatch, *Value-Freedom in Science and Technology*; Veatch, "Consensus of Expertise"; and Veatch, "Technology Assessment."

2. Beauchamp and Childress, *Principles of Biomedical Ethics*, 5th ed.; and Gillon, *Principles of Health Care Ethics*.

3. National Commission for the Protection of Human Subjects of Biomedical and Behavioral Research, *Belmont Report*.

4. Freedman, "Equipoise and the Ethics of Clinical Research"; and Veatch, "Indifference of Subjects"; Miller and Veatch, "Symposium on Equipoise."

5. Mill, "Utilitarianism," ch. 5, 418–34.

6. Pellegrino and Thomasma, *For the Patient's Good*.

7. Ibid., 81.

8. Ibid., 21–22, 45–46.

9. Engelhardt, *Foundations of Bioethics*, 2nd ed., 103–31 and passim; cf. Engelhardt, *Foundations of Bioethics*, 66ff.

10. Engelhardt, *Foundations of Bioethics*, 84, 336.

11. Brody, *Life and Death Decision Making*.

12. Ibid., 35–42.

13. Ibid., 17–22, cf., 32–35.

14. Ibid., 76–77.

15. Ibid., 22–32.

16. Ibid., 42–48.

17. Ross, *Foundations of Ethics*; and Ross, *Right and the Good*.

18. Ross, *Right and the Good*, 21.

19. Published in 1981 as Veatch, *Theory of Medical Ethics*.

20. Beauchamp, "Reply to Rachels," 67–75; cf. Beauchamp, *Intending Death*.

21. Elsewhere I have long held that people known to be permanently unconscious are more appropriately classified as deceased and therefore cannot be killed. See Veatch, "Whole-Brain-Oriented Concept of Death."

22. Smith, "Origin and Uses of *Primum non nocere*"; and Ross, *Right and the Good*, 21.

23. Clouser and Gert, "Critique of Principlism"; Green, Gert, and Clouser, "Method of Public Morality versus the Method of Principlism"; Clouser and Gert, "Morality vs. Principlism"; and Clouser, "Common Morality as an Alternative to Principlism."

24. Gert, Culver, and Clouser, *Bioethics* (1997), 34; and Gert, Culver, and Clouser, *Bioethics* (2006), 36.

25. Veatch, "Contract and the Critique of Principlism."

26. Rawls, *Theory of Justice*, 42–44.

27. See, for example, Gert, Culver, and Clouser, *Bioethics* (1997), 5, 9, 21, 76.

28. Gert, Culver, and Clouser, *Bioethics* (2006), 10.

29. Ibid., 11.

30. Gert, Culver, and Clouser, *Bioethics* (1997), 25.

31. Ibid., 32, 80.

32. The members are identified by title and not academic degree so establishing the academic discipline of each member is difficult. Most, however, identify with faculties outside of medicine.

33. For example, as we have seen Engelhardt, Gert, and utilitarians all explicitly reject a separate and independent principle of justice.

BIBLIOGRAPHY

The Gifford Lectures: History and Previous Lectures

Barth, Karl. *The Knowledge of God and the Service of God According to the Teaching of the Reformation, Recalling the Scottish Confession of 1560*. London: Hodder and Stoughton, [1938]. References are to the 1955 third impression.

Dewey, John. *The Quest for Certainty*. New York: Minton Balch, 1929.

Gifford, Adam. "Trust, Disposition and Settlement of the late Adam Gifford, Sometime One of the Senators of the College of Justice, Scotland, dated 21st August, 1885," in *Lord Gifford and His Lectures: A Centenary Retrospect*, edited by Stanley L. Jaki, 66–76. Edinburgh: Scottish Academic Press, 1986.

Hauerwas, Stanley. *With the Grain of the Universe: The Church's Witness and Natural Theology*. Grand Rapids, MI: Brazos Press, 2001.

Jaki, Stanley L. *Lord Gifford and His Lectures: A Centenary Retrospect*. Edinburgh: Scottish Academic Press, 1986.

James, William. *The Varieties of Religious Experience: A Study in Human Nature*. New York: Longmans, Green, and Co., 1902.

Jones, Bernard E. "The Concept of Natural Theology in the Gifford Lectures." Unpublished doctoral diss., University of Leeds, May 1966.

———, ed. *Earnest Enquirers after Truth: A Gifford Anthology; Excerpts from Gifford Lectures 1888–1968*. London: Allen & Unwin, 1970.

MacIntyre, Alasdair. *Three Rival Versions of Moral Enquiry: Encyclopedia, Genealogy, and Tradition*. Notre Dame, IN: University of Notre Dame Press, 1990.

Murdoch, Iris. *Metaphysics as a Guide to Morals*. New York: Penguin, 1994.

Niebuhr, Reinhold. *The Nature and Destiny of Man: A Christian Interpretation*, 2 vols. Louisville, KY: Westminster John Knox, 1996.

O'Neill, Onora. *Autonomy and Trust in Bioethics*. Cambridge: Cambridge University Press, 2002.

Perry, Ralph Barton. *Realms of Value*. Cambridge, MA: Harvard University Press, 1954, 90.

Ross, W. D. *Foundations of Ethics*. Oxford: Oxford University Press, 1939.

Tillich, Paul. *Systematic Theology*, 3 vols. Chicago: University of Chicago Press, 1967.

Whitehead, Alfred North. *Process and Reality*, corrected ed. Edited by David Ray Griffin and Donald W. Sherburne. New York: Free Press, 1979.

Witham, Larry. *The Measure of God: Our Century-Long Struggle to Reconcile Science & Religion: The Story of the Gifford Lectures*. New York: Harper-Collins, 2005.

Other Sources

Adams, Francis. *The Genuine Works of Hippocrates Translated from the Greek with a Preliminary Discourse and Annotations*, 2 vols. London: Sydenham Society, 1849.

American Medical Association (AMA). *Code of Medical Ethics: Adopted by the American Medical Association at Philadelphia, May, 1847, and by the New York Academy of Medicine in October, 1847*. New York: H. Ludwig and Company, 1848.

———. *Current Opinions of the Council on Ethical and Judicial Affairs of the American Medical Association: Including the Principles of Medical Ethics and Rules of the Council on Ethical and Judicial Affairs*. Chicago: American Medical Association, 1989.

———. *Current Opinions of the Judicial Council of the American Medical Association*. Chicago: American Medical Association, 1981.

———. "Principles of Medical Ethics of the American Medical Association." *Journal of the American Medical Association* 164 (1957): 1119–20.

American Medical Association, Council on Ethical and Judicial Affairs (AMA, CEJA). *Code of Medical Ethics: Current Opinions with Annotations*. Chicago: American Medical Association, 1994.

———. *Code of Medical Ethics: Current Opinions with Annotations, 2006–2007*. Chicago: AMA Press, 2006.

———. *Code of Medical Ethics: Current Opinions with Annotations, 2008–2009*. Chicago: AMA Press, 2008.

———. *Code of Medical Ethics: Current Opinions with Annotations, 2010–2011*. Chicago: AMA Press, 2010.

————. "Physician Participation in Capital Punishment." *Journal of the American Medical Association* 270, no. 3 (July 21, 1993): 365–68.

Annas, George J., and Michael A., Grodin, eds. *The Nazi Doctors and the Nuremberg Code: Nuremberg Code: Human Rights in Human Experimentation*. New York: Oxford University Press, 1992.

Aquinas, Thomas. *Summa theologica*, edited by Fathers of the English Dominican Province. London: R & T Washbourne, Ltd. 1915.

Ashcroft, Richard. "Equipoise, Knowledge and Ethics in Clinical Research and Practice." *Bioethics* 13, no. 3–4 (1999): 314–26.

Baker, Robert. "The Historical Context of the American Medical Association's 1847 Code of Ethics." In *The Codification of Medical Morality: Historical and Philosophical Studies of the Formalization of Western Medical Morality in the Eighteenth and Nineteenth Centuries*. Volume 2, *Anglo-American Medical Ethics and Medical Jurisprudence in the Nineteenth Century*, edited by Robert Baker, 47–63. Dordrecht, Netherlands: Kluwer Academic Publishers, 1995. First published 1808.

Baker, Robert B., Arthur L. Caplan, Linda L. Emanuel, and Stephen R. Latham. *The American Medical Ethics Revolution: How the AMA's Code of Ethics Has Transformed Physicians' Relations to Patients, Professionals, and Society*. Baltimore: Johns Hopkins University Press, 1999.

Baker, Robert C., and Ehlke, Roland Cap, eds. *Natural Law: A Lutheran Reappraisal*. St. Louis: Concordia Publishing House, 2011.

Barth, Karl. *Church Dogmatics*, III/4. Translated by A. T. Mackay, et al., Edinburgh: T & T Clark, 1961.

Barth, Karl. *Ethics*. Edited by Dietrich Braun, translated by Geoffrey W. Bromiley. New York: Seabury Press, 1981.

Beauchamp, Tom L. "A Defense of the Common Morality." *Kennedy Institute of Ethics Journal* 13 (September 2003): 259–74.

————, ed. *Intending Death: The Ethics of Assisted Suicide and Euthanasia*. Upper Saddle River, NJ: Prentice Hall, 1996.

————. "A Reply to Rachels on Active and Passive Euthanasia." In *Social Ethics: Morality and Social Policy*, edited by T. A. Mappes and J. S. Zembaty, 67–75. New York: McGraw-Hill, 1977.

Beauchamp, Tom L., and James F. Childress. *Principles of Biomedical Ethics*, 4th ed. New York: Oxford University Press, 1994.

————. *Principles of Biomedical Ethics*, 5th ed. New York: Oxford University Press, 2001.

Beecher, Henry K. "Ethics and Clinical Research." *New England Journal of Medicine* 274 (1966): 1354–60.

Bell, John. "Introduction to the Code of Medical Ethics." In *The Codification of Medical Morality*, edited by Robert Baker, 65–72. Dordrecht, Netherlands: Kluwer Academic Publishers, 1995. First published 1847.

Berman, Harold Joseph. *Faith and Order: The Reconciliation of Law and Religion*. Grand Rapids, MI: Eerdmans, 1993.

Bernardin, Joseph A. Cardinal. *The Seamless Garment: Writings on the Consistent Ethic of Life*. Maryknoll, NY: Orbis Books, 2008.

The Book of Discipline of the United Methodist Church—2004. Nashville: United Methodist Publishing House, 2004.

Brandt, Richard B. *Ethical Theory: The Problems of Normative and Critical Ethics*. Englewood Cliffs, NJ: Prentice Hall, 1959.

Brock, Lord. "Euthanasia." *Proceedings of the Royal Society of Medicine*, July 1970, 661–63.

Brody, Baruch. *Life and Death Decision Making*. New York: Oxford University Press, 1988.

Brody, Howard, and Franklin G. Miller. "The Internal Morality of Medicine; Explication and Application to Managed Care." *Journal of Medicine and Philosophy* 23 (1998): 384–410.

Burgio, G. Roberto, and John D. Lantos, eds. *Primum non nocere Today*. Amsterdam: Elsevier, 1998.

Burns, C. R. "Reciprocity in the Development of Anglo-American Medical Ethics 1765–1865." In *Legacies in Ethics and Medicine*, edited by Chester R. Burns, 300–306. New York: Science History Publications, 1977.

Cabot, Richard C. "The Use of Truth and Falsehood in Medicine: An Experimental Study." *American Medicine* 5 (1903): 344–49.

Callahan, Daniel. "On Feeding the Dying." *Hastings Center Report* 13, no. 5 (1983): 22.

Caplan, Arthur. "The Ethics of Evil: The Challenge of the Lessons of the Nazi Medical Experiments." In *Dark Medicine: Rationalizing Medical Research*, edited by William R. LaFleur, Gernot Böhme, Susumu Shimazono, 63–72. Bloomington: Indiana University Press, 2007.

Carey, E. J. "The Formal Use of the Hippocratic Oath for Medical Students at Commencement Exercises." *Bulletin of the Association of American Medical Colleges* 3 (1928): 159–66.

Carrick, Paul. *Medical Ethics in Antiquity: Philosophical Perspectives on Abortion and Euthanasia.* Dordrecht, Holland: D. Reidel Publishing, 1985.

Cassell, Eric J. *The Healer's Art.* Cambridge, MA: MIT Press, 1985.

"Central Ethical Committee." *British Medical Journal Supplement,* May 1, 1971, 30.

Childress, James F., Eric M. Meslin, and Harold T. Shapiro, eds. *Belmont Revisited: Ethical Principles for Research with Human Subjects.* Washington, DC: Georgetown University Press, 2005.

Clouser, K. Danner. "Common Morality as an Alternative to Principlism." *Kennedy Institute of Ethics Journal* 5 (1995): 219–36.

Clouser, K. Danner, and Bernard Gert. "A Critique of Principlism." *Journal of Medicine and Philosophy* 15, no. 2 (April 1990): 219–36.

———. "Morality vs. Principlism." In *Principles of Health Care Ethics,* edited by Raanan Gillon, 251–66. New York: Wiley, 1994.

[Commission for Visiting the Universities and Colleges in Scotland]. *Evidence, Oral and Documentary, Taken and Received by the Commissioners Appointed by His Majesty George IV, July 23d, 1826; and Re-appointed by His Majesty, William IV, October 12th, 1830; for Visiting the Universities of Scotland,* Vol. 1. *University of Edinburgh.* London: W. Clowes and Sones, Stamford Street, for His Majesty's Stationery Office, 1837.

Coxe, John Redman. *The Writings of Hippocrates and Galen. Epitomised from the Original Latin.* Philadelphia: Lindsay and Blakiston, 1846.

Dalzel, Andrew. *History of the University of Edinburgh from Its Foundation.* 2 vols. Edinburgh: Edmonston and Douglas, 1862.

Daniels, Norman. *Just Health Care.* Cambridge: Cambridge University Press, 1985.

Daniels, Norman, and James E. Sabin. *Setting Limits Fairly: Can We Learn to Share Medical Resources?* New York: Oxford University Press, 2002.

DeGrazia, David. "Common Morality, Coherence, and the Principles of Biomedical Ethics." *Kennedy Institute of Ethics Journal* 13 (September 2003): 219–30.

———. "Grounding a Right to Health Care in Self-Respect and Self-Esteem." *Public Affairs Quarterly* 5 (October 1991): 301–18.

Donaldson, D. J. *Do No Harm.* New York: Jove Books, 1999.

Edelstein, Ludwig. "The Hippocratic Oath: Text, Translation and Interpretation." In *Ancient Medicine: Selected Papers of Ludwig Edelstein,* edited by

Owsei Temkin and C. Lilian Temkin, 3–64. Baltimore: Johns Hopkins University Press, 1967.

Engelhardt, H. Tristram. *Bioethics and Secular Humanism: The Search for a Common Morality*. Philadelphia: Trinity Press International, 1991.

———. *The Foundations of Bioethics*. New York: Oxford University Press, 1986.

———. *The Foundations of Bioethics*, 2nd ed. New York: Oxford University Press, 1996.

———. *The Foundations of Christian Bioethics*. Lisse, Netherlands: Swets & Zeitlinger Publishers, 2000.

Firth, Roderick. "Ethical Absolutism and the Ideal Observer Theory." *Philosophy and Phenomenological Research* 12 (1952): 317–45.

Fletcher, Joseph. *Morals and Medicine*. Boston: Beacon Press, 1960.

Frankel, Lorry R., Amnon Goldworth, Mary V. Rorty, and William A. Silverman, eds. *Ethical Dilemmas in Pediatrics: Cases and Commentaries*. New York: Cambridge University Press, 2005.

Freedman, Benjamin. "Equipoise and the Ethics of Clinical Research." *New England Journal of Medicine* 317 (1987): 141–45.

Friedlander, Walter J. "Oaths Given by US and Canadian Medical Schools, 1977: Profession of Medical Values." *Social Sciences and Medicine* 16 (1982): 115–20.

Galvao-Sobrinho, Carlos R. "Hippocratic Ideals, Medical Ethics, and the Practice of Medicine in the Early Middle Ages: The Legacy of the Hippocratic Oath." *Journal of the History of Medicine* 51 (October 1996): 438–55.

Garzya, Antonio. "Science et conscience dans la pratique medicale de l'antiquite tardive et byzantine." In *Medecine et morale dans l'antiquite*, edited by Hellmut Flashar and Jacques Jouana, 337–63. Geneve: Fondation Hardt, 1997.

"General Medical Council: Disciplinary Committee." *British Medical Journal Supplement*, no. 3442, March 20, 1971, 79–80.

Gert, Bernard. *Common Morality: Deciding What to Do*. New York: Oxford University Press, 2004.

Gert, Bernard. Charles M. Culver, and K. Danner Clouser. *Bioethics: A Return to Fundamentals*. New York: Oxford University Press, 1997.

———. *Bioethics: A Systematic Approach*. New York: Oxford University Press, 2006.

———. "Common Morality versus Specified Principlism: Reply to Richardson." *Journal of Medicine and Philosophy* 25, no. 3 (2000): 308–22.

Gifford, Fred. "Community-Equipoise and the Ethics of Randomized Clinical Trials." *Bioethics* 9, no. 2 (1995): 127–48.

Gillon, Raanan, ed. *Principles of Health Care Ethics*. New York: Wiley, 1994.

Gordon, Theodore, Herbert Gerjuoy, and Mark Anderson, eds. *Life-Extending Technologies: A Technology Assessment*. New York: Pergamon Press, 1979.

Green, Ronald M. "Health Care and Justice in Contract Theory Perspective." In *Ethics and Health Policy*, edited by Robert M. Veatch and Roy Branson, 111–26. Cambridge, MA: Ballinger Publishing Company, 1976.

Green, Ronald M., Bernard Gert, and K. Danner Clouser. "The Method of Public Morality versus the Method of Principlism." *Journal of Medicine and Philosophy* 18, no. 5 (October 1993): 477–89.

Gregory, John. *Lectures on the Duties and Qualifications of a Physician*. London: W. Strahan and T. Cadell, in the Strand, 1772.

Gregory of Nazianzus. "Oration VII: Panegyric on His Brother S. Caesarius." In *The Nicene and Post-Nicene Fathers*, vol. VII, edited by P. Schaff and H. Wace, 229–38. Grand Rapids, MI: Eerdmans, n.d.

Gunter, W. Stephen, Scott J. Jones, Ted A. Campbell, Rebekah Miles, and Randy Maddox. *Wesley and the Quadrilateral: Renewing the Conversation*. Nashville: Abingdon, 1997.

Habbi, Joseph. "L'eredita Ippocratica dell'obligo morale nella medicina araba." *Medicina Nei Secoli* 7 (1995): 79–93

———. "Le role de Hunayn, medecin et traducteur." *Medicini Nei Secoli* 6 (1994): 293–308.

Hamel, Ronald P., and James J. Walter, eds. *Artificial Nutrition and Hydration and the Permanently Unconscious Patient: The Catholic Debate*. Washington, DC: Georgetown University Press, 2007.

Haring, Bernard. *Medical Ethics*. Fides Publishers, Inc., 1973.

Harrell, David Edwin. *Oral Roberts: An American Life*. Bloomington: Indiana University Press, 1985.

Hauerwas, Stanley. *Suffering Presence: Theological Reflection on Medicine, the Mentally Handicapped, and the Church*. Notre Dame, IN: University of Notre Dame Press, 1986.

Hayflick, Leonard. "Theories of Biological Aging." *Experimental Gerontology* 20 (1985): 145–59.

Healy, Edwin F. *Medical Ethics*. Chicago: Loyola University Press, 1956.

Hoffding, Harold. *A History of Modern Philosophy: A Sketch of the History of Philosophy from the Close of the Renaissance to Our Own Day*. London: Macmillan, 1908.

Hutcheson, Francis. *Illustrations on the Moral Sense*. Cambridge, MA: Belknap Press of Harvard University Press, 1971. First published 1728.

Inman, T. *Foundation for a New Theory and Practice of Medicine*. London: John Churchill, 1860.

Irish, Donald P., and Daniel W. McMurry. "Professional Oaths and American Medical Colleges." *Journal of Chronic Diseases* 18 (1965): 275–89.

Jacquart, Danielle. 1994. "Le sens donné par Constantin l'Africain à son oeuvre: les chapitres introductifs en arabe et en latin." In *Constantine the African and 'Ali ibn al-Abbas al-Magusi: The Pantegni and Related Texts*, edited by C. Burnett and D. Jacquart, 71–89. Leyde: E. J. Brill.

James, William. *Essays in Radical Empiricism*. New York: Longmans, Green, and Co., 1912.

Jerome, "Letter LII," in *The Nicene and Post-Nicene Fathers*, vol. VI, edited by P. Schaff and H. Wace, 89–96. Grand Rapids, MI: Eerdmans, 1954.

Johnson, Allen, and Dumas Malone. *Dictionary of American Biography*, vol. 4. New York: Scribner's, 1957.

Jones, James H. *Bad Blood: The Tuskegee Syphilis Experiment*, new and exp. ed. New York: Free Press; 1993.

Jones, W. H. S. *The Doctor's Oath: An Essay in the History of Medicine*. Cambridge: University Press, 1924.

Jonsen, Albert R. "Do No Harm." *Annals of Internal Medicine* 88 (1978): 827–32.

Jonsen, Albert, R., Mark Siegler, and William Winslade. *Clinical Ethics: A Practical Approach to Ethical Decisions in Clinical Medicine*. New York: McGraw Hill, 2010.

Jouanna, Jacques. "La lecture de l'éthiquee Hippocratique chez Galien." In *Medecine et morale dans l'antiquite*, edited by Hellmut Flashar and Jacques Jouana, 211–53. Geneve: Fondation Hardt, 1997.

Kant, Immanuel. "On the Supposed Right to Tell Lies from Benevolent Motives," translated by Thomas Kingsmill Abbott and reprinted in Kant's *Critique of Practical Reason and Other Works on the Theory of Ethics*, 361–65. London: Longmans, 1909. First published 1797.

Kappa Lambda. "Formula to Be Observed at the Initiation of a Member Elect, Together with the Address to Be Delivered on This Occasion." Unpublished manuscript, ca. 1824–26.

———. *Constitution and By-Laws*. Philadelphia: Kappa Lambda, 1825.

Karlawish, Jason H. T., and John Lantos. "Community Equipoise and the Architecture of Clinical Research," *Cambridge Quarterly of Healthcare Ethics* 6 (1997): 385–96.

Kelly, Gerald. *Medico-Moral Problems*. St. Louis: Catholic Hospital Association, 1958.

Kevorkian, Jack. *Prescription Medicide: The Goodness of Planned Death*. Buffalo, NY: Prometheus Books, 1991.

Kudlien, Fridolf. "Medical Ethics and Popular Ethics in Greece and Rome." *Clio Medica* 5 (1970): 91–121.

Lambeth Conference. *Encyclical Letter from the Bishops, with Resolutions and Reports Publication Information*. New York: Macmillan [1930].

Lammers, Stephen E., and Allen Verhey, eds. *On Moral Medicine: Theological Perspectives in Medical Ethics*. Grand Rapids, MI: Eerdmans, 1987.

Larijani, Bagher, and Farzaneh Zahedi. 2006. "An Introductory on Medical Ethics History in Different Era in Iran." *Daru*, Supplement #1 (2006): 10–16.

Larkey, Sanford V. "The Hippocratic Oath in Elizabethan England." *Bulletin of the History of Medicine* 4 (1936): 201–19.

Levey, Martin. *Medical Ethics of Medieval Islam with Special Reference to Al-Ruhawi's "Practical Ethics of the Physician."* Philadelphia: American Philosophical Society, 1967.

Lief, Harold I., and Renée C. Fox. "Training for 'Detached Concern' in Medical Students." In *The Psychological Basis of Medical Practice*, edited by Victor F. Lief and Nina R. Lief, 12–35. New York: Hoeber Medical Division of Harper and Row, 1963.

Lifton, Robert J. *Nazi Doctors*. New York: Basic Books, 1986.

Lindsay, Ronald A. "Slaves, Embryos, and Nonhuman Animals: Moral Status and the Limitations of Common Morality Theory." *Kennedy Institute of Ethics Journal* 15, no. 4 (December 2005): 323–46.

MacKinney, Loren C. "Medical Ethics and Etiquette in the Early Middle Ages." *Bulletin of the History of Medicine* 26 (1952): 1–31.

Maclean, Ian. *The Renaissance Notion of Woman: A Study in the Fortunes of Scholasticism and Medieval Science in European Intellectual Life*. Cambridge: Cambridge University Press, 1985.

Matthai, Georg. *"Tractatus de philosophia medici sive . . .* Hippocratis Coi liber de honestate, etc., etc.," Gottingae 1740, cited in Kudlien, Fridolf, "Medical

Ethics and Popular Ethics in Greece and Rome," *Clio Medica* 5 (1970): 91–121.

McCormick, Richard A. *Health and Medicine in the Catholic Tradition.* New York: Crossroad Publishing, 1984.

McFadden, Charles J. *Medical Ethics*, 6th ed. Philadelphia: F. A. Davis. 1967.

McLean, Sheila. *First Do No Harm: Law, Ethics and Healthcare.* Burlington, VT: Ashgate, 2006.

Medical Association of the District of Columbia. *Regulations and System of Ethics of the Medical Association of Washington.* Washington, DC: Barron, 1833.

Medical Society of the State of New York. *A System of Medical Ethics.* New York: Grattan, 1823.

Medico–Chirurgical Society of Baltimore. *A System of Medical Ethics.* Baltimore: James Lucas and E. K. Deaver, 1832.

Mehlman, Maxwell J. *Wondergenes: Genetic Enhancement and the Future of Society.* Bloomington: Indiana University Press, 2003.

Meilaender, Gilbert. "On Removing Food and Water: Against the Stream." *Hastings Center Report* 14, no. 6 (1984): 11–13.

Meyer, Bernard C. "Truth and the Physician." In *Ethical Issues in Medicine*, edited by E. Fuller Torrey, 159–77. Boston: Little, Brown, 1968.

Miles, Steven H. *The Hippocratic Oath and the Ethics of Medicine.* New York: Oxford University Press, 2004.

Mill, John Stuart. "Utilitarianism." In *Ethical Theories: A Book of Readings*, edited by A. I. Melden, 391–434. Englewood Cliffs, NJ: Prentice Hall, 1967.

Miller, Franklin G., and Howard Brody. "A Critique of Clinical Equipoise." *Hastings Center Report* 33, no. 3 (2003): 19–28.

———. "Professional Integrity and Physician-Assisted Death." *Hastings Center Report* 25, no. 3 (May–June 1995): 8–17.

Miller, Franklin G., and Robert M. Veatch, eds. "Symposium on Equipoise and the Ethics of Clinical Trials." *Journal of Medicine and Philosophy* 32 (2007).

Morison, Robert S. "Rights and Responsibilities: Redressing the Uneasy Balance." *Hastings Center Report* 4, no. 2 (1974): 1–4.

National Commission for the Protection of Human Subjects of Biomedical and Behavioral Research. *The Belmont Report: Ethical Principles and Guidelines for the Protection of Human Subjects of Research.* Washington, DC: US Government Printing Office, 1978.

Novack, Dennis H., Barbara J. Detering, Robert Arnold, Morissa Ladinsky, and John C. Pezzullo. "Physician's Attitudes toward Using Deception to Resolve

Difficult Ethical Problems." *Journal of the American Medical Association* 261, no. 20 (May 26, 1989): 2980–85.

Oken, Donald. "What to Tell Cancer Patients: A Study of Medical Attitudes." *Journal of the American Medical Association* 175 (April 1, 1961): 1120–28.

O'Rourke, Kevin D., and Philip Boyle. *Medical Ethics: Sources of Catholic Teachings*. St. Louis: Catholic Health Association, 1989.

Orr, Robert D., Norman Pang, Edmund D. Pellegrino, and Mark Siegler. "Use of the Hippocratic Oath: A Review of Twentieth Century Practice and a Content Analysis of Oaths Administered in Medical Schools in the US and Canada in 1993." *Journal of Clinical Ethics* 8 (1997): 377–88.

Paul, Charlotte. "Internal and External Morality of Medicine: Lessons from New Zealand." *British Medical Journal* 320 (February 19, 2000): 499–503.

Pellegrino, Edmund D. "The Goals and Ends of Medicine: How Are They to Be Defined?" In *The Goals of Medicine: The Forgotten Issue in Health Care Reform*, edited by Mark J. Hanson and Daniel Callahan, 55–68. Washington, DC: Georgetown University Press, 1999.

———. "The Internal Morality of Clinical Medicine: A Paradigm for the Ethics of the Helping and Healing Professions." *Journal of Medicine and Philosophy* 26, no. 6 (2001): 559–79.

Pellegrino, Edmund D., and David C. Thomasma. *For the Patient's Good: The Restoration of Beneficence in Health Care*. New York: Oxford University Press, 1988.

Percival, Thomas. *Medical Ethics; or, a Code of Institutes and Precepts, Adapted to the Professional Conduct of Physicians and Surgeons; To which Is Added an Appendix; Containing a Discourse on Hospital Duties; [by Rev. Thomas Bassnett Percival, LL.B.] and Notes and Illustrations*. Manchester: S. Russell, for J. Johnson, St. Paul's Church Yard, and R. Bicherstaff, Strand, London, 1803.

———. *Medical Jurisprudence; Or, a Code of Ethics and Institutes, Adapted to the Professions of Physic and Surgery*. [Manchester, 1794].

———. *Moral and Literary Dissertations, on the Following Subjects: 1. On Truth and Faithfulness. 2. On Habit and Association. 3. On Inconsistency of Expertation in Literary Pursuits. 4. On a Taste for the General Beauties of Nature. 5. On a Taste for the Fine Arts. 6. On the Alliance of Natural History, and Philosophy, with Poetry. To which Are Added a Tribute to the Memory of Charles de Polier, Esq. and an Appendix*. Warrington: W. Eyres, for J. Johnson, London: 1784.

[————]. *Philosophical, Medical, and Experimental Essays . . . to which Is Added an Appendix; Containing a Letter to the Author from Dr. Saunders, on the Solution of Human Calculi*. London: J. Johnson, 1776.

————. *The Works, Literary, Moral, and Philosophical, of Thomas Percival; to which Are Prefixed, Memoirs of His Life and Writings, and a Selection from His Literary Correspondence. A New Edition*. 2 vols., edited by Edward Percival. Bath: Richard Cruttwell for J. Johnson, St. Paul's Church-yard, London, 1807.

Perry, Ralph Barton. *The Thought and Character of William James, as Revealed in Unpublished Correspondence and Notes, Together with His Published Writings*. Boston: Little, Brown, 1935.

Porter, Jean. *Ministers of the Law: A Natural Law Theory of Legal Authority*. Grand Rapids, MI: Eerdmans, 2010.

————. *Natural and Divine Law: Reclaiming the Tradition for Christian Ethics*. Grand Rapids, MI: Eerdmans, 1999.

————. *Nature as Reason: A Thomistic Theory of the Natural Law*. Grand Rapids, MI: Eerdmans, 2005.

Prioreschi, Plinio. "The Hippocratic Oath: A Code for Physicians, not a Pythagorean Manifesto. *Medical Hypotheses* 44 (1995): 447–62.

Rawls, John. *A Theory of Justice*. Cambridge, MA: Harvard University Press, 1971.

Roberts, Oral. *Expect a Miracle: My Life and Ministry; An Autobiography*. Nashville: Thomas Nelson, 1995.

Rosner, Fred. "The Life of Moses Maimonides, a Prominent Medieval Physician." *Einstein Quarterly Journal of Biology and Medicine* 19 (2002): 125–28.

————. *The Medical Legacy of Moses Maimonides*. Hoboken, NJ: KTAV Publishing House, 1998.

————. "Organ Transplantation in Jewish Law." In *Jewish Bioethics*, edited by Fred Rosner and J. David Bleich, 358–74. New York: Sanhedrin Press, 1979.

Ross, W. D. *The Right and the Good*. Oxford: Oxford University Press, 1930.

Roth, Russell B. "Medicine's Ethical Responsibilities." *Journal of the American Medical Association* 215 (1971): 1956–68.

Rozenberg, Joseph J., ed. *Bioethical and Ethical Issues Surrounding the Trials and Code of Nuremberg: Nuremberg Revisited*. Lewiston, NY: Edwin Mellen Press, 2003.

Russo, Michael P. "Recommendations for the Ethical Use of Pharmacologic Fatigue Countermeasures in the US Military." *Aviation, Space, and Environmental Medicine* 78, no. 5, sec. 2, suppl. (2007): B119–27.

Sacred Congregation for the Doctrine of the Faith. *Declaration on Euthanasia.* Rome: Sacred Congregation for the Doctrine of the Faith, May 5, 1980.

Sandulescu, C. "*Primum non nocere*: Philological Commentaries on a Medical Aphorism." *Acta antiqua hungarica* 13 (1965): 359–68.

Sandys, John Edwin. *A History of Classical Scholarship.* 3 vols. New York: Hafner Publishing Co., 1967. First published 1921.

Savulescu, Julian, and Nick Bostrom, eds. *Human Enhancement.* Oxford: Oxford University Press, 2009.

Schleiner, Winfried. *Medical Ethics in the Renaissance.* Washington, DC: Georgetown University Press, 1995.

Shock, Nathan W. "The Physiological Basis of Aging." *Frontiers in Medicine— Implications for the Future,* edited by Robert J. Morin and Richard J. Bing, 300–12. New York: Human Sciences Press, 1985.

Smith, Adam. *The Theory of Moral Sentiments,* edited by D. D. Raphael and A. L. Macfie. Indianapolis: Liberty Classics, 1976. First published 1759.

Smith, Cedric M. "Origin and Uses of *Primum non nocere*—Above All, Do No Harm!" *Journal of Clinical Pharmacology* 45 (2005): 371–77.

Smith, Wesley D. *The Hippocratic Tradition.* Ithaca, NY: Cornell University Press, 1979.

Strohmaier, Gotthard. "Hunayn Ibn Ishaq et le serment d'Hippocrate." *Arabica* 21, no. 3 (1974): 318–23.

Sulmasy, Daniel P. "Terri Schiavo and the Roman Catholic Tradition of Forgoing Extraordinary Means of Care." *Journal of Law, Medicine & Ethics* 33 (Summer 2005): 359–62.

Temkin, Owsei. *Hippocrates in a World of Pagans and Christians.* Baltimore: Johns Hopkins University Press, 1991.

Tendler, M. D. "Cessation of Brain Function: Ethical Implications in Terminal Care and Organ Transplant." In *Brain Death: Interrelated Medical and Social Issues,* edited by Julius Korein, 394–97. New York: New York Academy of Sciences, 1978.

Thorsen, Don. *The Wesleyan Quadrilateral: Scripture, Tradition, Reason and Experience as a Model of Evangelical Theology.* Grand Rapids, MI: Zondervan, 1990.

Todd, James S. "Report of the Ad Hoc Committee on the Principles of Medical Ethics [of the American Medical Association]." Unpublished report, 1979.

Tollefsen, Christopher, ed. *Artificial Nutrition and Hydration: The New Catholic Debate*. Dordrecht, Netherlands: Springer, 2010.

Turner, Leigh. "Bioethics in a Multicultural World: Medicine and Morality in Pluralistic Settings." *Health Care Analysis: An International Journal of Health Philosophy and Policy* 11, no. 2 (June 2003): 99–117.

———. "Zones of Consensus and Zones of Conflict: Questioning the 'Common Morality' Presumption in Bioethics." *Kennedy Institute of Ethics Journal* 13, no. 3 (September 2003): 193–218.

United States Conference of Catholic Bishops. "Catholic Campaign to End the Use of the Death Penalty." Washington, DC: USCCB, n.d.

———. *Ethical and Religious Directives for Catholic Health Care Services*. Washington, DC: USCCB, 2001.

US Public Health Service. "Final Report of the Tuskegee Syphilis Study ad hoc Advisory Panel." Washington, DC: US Government Printing Office, 1973.

Vandrunen, David. "The Context of Natural Law: John Calvin's Doctrine of the Two Kingdoms." *Journal of Church and State* 46, no. 3 (2004): 503–25.

Veatch, Robert M. "Benevolent Lies: Fallible Universalism and the Quest for an International Standard." *Formosan Journal of Medical Humanities* 7, no. 1 & 2 (June 2006): 3–18.

———. "Common Morality and Human Finitude: A Foundation for Bioethics." In *Weltanschaulilche Offenheit in der Bioethik*, edited by Eva Baumann, Alexander Bink, Arnd T. May, Peter Schroder, and Corinna Iris Schutzeiechel, 37–50. Berlin: Duncker & Humblot, 2004.

———. "Consensus of Expertise: The Role of Consensus of Experts in Formulating Public Policy and Estimating Facts." *Journal of Medicine and Philosophy* 16 (1991): 427–45.

———. "Contract and the Critique of Principlism: Hypothetical Contract as Epistemological Theory and as Method of Conflict Resolution." In *Building Bioethics: Conversations with Clouser and Friends on Medical Ethics*, edited by Loretta M. Kopelman, 121–43. Dordrecht, Netherlands: Kluwer Academic Publishers, 1999.

———. *Disrupted Dialogue: Medical Ethics and the Collapse of Physician/ Humanist Communication (1770–1980)*. New York: Oxford University Press, 2005.

————. *The Foundations of Justice: Why the Retarded and the Rest of Us Have Claims to Equality.* New York: Oxford University Press, 1986.

————. "Generalization of Expertise: Scientific Expertise and Value Judgments." *Hastings Center Studies* 1, no. 2 (1973): 29–40.

————. "The Hippocratic Ethic: Consequentialism, Individualism and Paternalism." In *No Rush to Judgment—Essays on Medical Ethics,* edited by David H. Smith and Linda M. Bernstein, 238–65. Bloomington: Poynter Center, Indiana University, 1978.

————. "Human Experimentation—Ethical Questions Persist." *Hastings Center Report* 3, no. 3 (June 1973): 1–3.

————. "The Impossibility of a Morality Internal to Medicine." *Journal of Medicine and Philosophy* 26 (2001): 621–64.

————. "Indifference of Subjects: An Alternative to Equipoise in Randomized Clinical Trials." *Social Philosophy & Policy* 19, no. 2 (2002): 295–323.

————. "The Irrelevance of Equipoise." *Journal of Medicine and Philosophy* 32 (2007): 167–83.

————. "Is There a Common Morality?" *Kennedy Institute of Ethics Journal* 13 (September 2003): 189–92.

————. "Nazis and Hippocratists: Searching for the Moral Relation." *Psychohistory Review* 16 (Fall 1987): 15–31.

————. *Patient, Heal Thyself.* New York: Oxford University Press, 2009.

————. "Statement of Robert Veatch, PhD, Hastings Institute, Hastings-on-Hudson, NY." In *Quality of Health Care—Human Experimentation, 1973: Hearings before the Subcommittee on Health of the Committee on Labor and Public Welfare, United States Senate, Ninety-Third Congress: First Session on S. 974, S. 878, S.J. Res. 71: Part I,* 265–75. Washington, DC: US Government Printing Office, February 21 and 22, 1973.

————. "Technology Assessment: Inevitably a Value Judgment." In *Getting Doctors to Listen: Ethics and Outcomes Data in Context,* edited by Philip J. Boyle, 180–95. Washington, DC: Georgetown University Press, 1998.

————. *A Theory of Medical Ethics.* New York: Basic Books, 1981.

————. *Value-Freedom in Science and Technology.* Missoula, MT: Scholars Press, 1976.

————. "The Whole-Brain-Oriented Concept of Death: An Outmoded Philosophical Formulation." *Journal of Thanatology* 3 (1975): 13–30.

Veatch, Robert M., and Cheryl C. Macpherson. "Medical School Oath-Taking: The Moral Controversy." *Journal of Clinical Ethics* 21, no. 4 (Winter 2010): 335–45.

Veatch, Robert M., and Carol G. Mason. "Hippocratic vs. Judeo-Christian Medical Ethics: Principles in Conflict." *Journal of Religious Ethics* 15 (Spring 1987): 86–105.

Veatch, Robert M., and William E. Stempsey. "Incommensurability: Its Implications for the Patient/Physician Relation." *Journal of Medicine and Philosophy* 20, no. 3 (June 1995): 253–69.

Verhey, Allen. "The Doctor's Oath—and a Christian Swearing It." *Linacre Quarterly* 15 (1984): 139–57.

von Staden, Heinrich. "'In a Pure and Holy Way': Personal and Professional Conduct in the Hippocratic Oath?" *Journal of the History of Medicine* 51 (October 1996): 404–37.

Walford, Roy. *Maximum Life Span.* New York: Norton, 1983.

Walsh, James F. *History of the Medical Society of the State of New York.* [Westbury]: Medical Society of the State of New York, 1907.

Warren, John, Lemuel Hayward, and John Fleet. "Boston Medical Police, Boston Medical Association." In *The Codification of Medical Morality: Historical and Philosophical Studies of the Formalization of Western Medical Morality in the Eighteenth and Nineteenth Centuries.* Vol. 2, *Anglo-American Medical Ethics and Medical Jurisprudence in the Nineteenth Century*, edited by Robert Baker, 41–46. Dordrecht, Netherlands: Kluwer Academic Publishers, 1995. First published 1808.

Weijer, Charles. "For and Against: Clinical Equipoise and Not the Uncertainty Principle Is the Moral Underpinning of the Randomised Controlled Trial." *British Medical Journal* 321 (September 23, 2000): 756–58.

[Wesley, John]. *Primitive Physick: or, An Easy and Natural Method of Curing Most Diseases.* London: Thomas Trye, 1747.

Woodhead, Avril D., Anthony D. Blackett, and Alexander Hollaender. *Molecular Biology of Aging.* New York: Plenum Press, 1985.

World Medical Association. "Declaration of Geneva." *World Medical Journal* 3 (1956): supplement, 10–12.

Zylinska, Joanna. "Playing God, Playing Adam: The Politics and Ethics of Enhancement." *Journal of Bioethical Inquiry*, no. 2 (June 2010): 149–61.

INDEX